T0319443

Making a Good Life

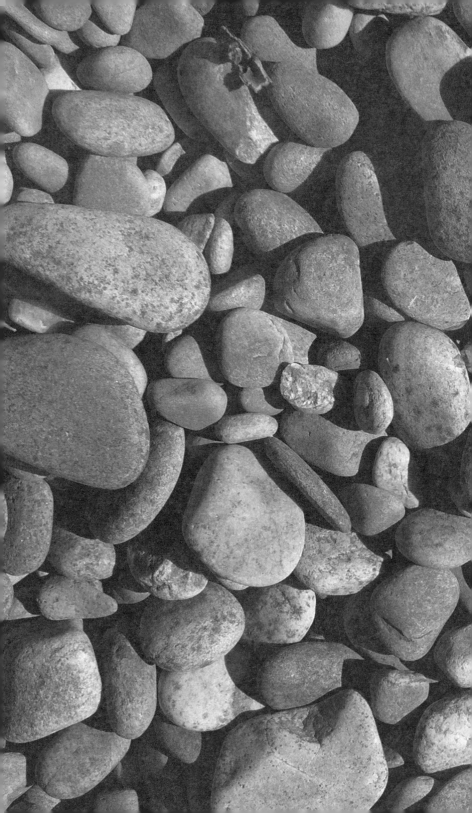

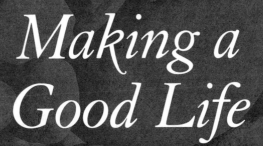

Making a Good Life

An Ethnography of Nature,
Ethics, and Reproduction

KATHARINE
DOW

PRINCETON UNIVERSITY PRESS
Princeton & Oxford

Copyright © 2016 by Princeton University Press

Published by Princeton University Press
41 William Street, Princeton, New Jersey 08540

In the United Kingdom: Princeton University Press
6 Oxford Street, Woodstock, Oxfordshire OX20 1TR

press.princeton.edu

Jacket art courtesy of iStock

Library of Congress Cataloging-in-Publication Data

Names: Dow, Katharine, 1982– author.
Title: Making a good life : an ethnography of nature, ethics,
and reproduction / Katharine Dow.
Description: Princeton : Princeton University Press, [2016] | Includes
bibliographical references and index.
Identifiers: LCCN 2015037390 | ISBN 9780691167480 (cloth : acid-free
paper) | ISBN 9780691171753 (pbk. : acid-free paper)
Subjects: LCSH: Human reproduction—Social aspects. | Anthropology.
Classification: LCC HQ766 .D68 2016 | DDC 301—dc23 LC record
available at http://lccn.loc.gov/2015037390

British Library Cataloging-in-Publication Data is available

This book has been composed in Granjon LT Std

Printed on acid-free paper. ∞

Printed in the United States of America

1 3 5 7 9 10 8 6 4 2

This book is dedicated to the future generations.

CONTENTS

ACKNOWLEDGEMENTS

My first and most obvious debt of gratitude goes to the residents of Spey Bay and the surrounding area who let me share their lives for the time I lived there. Living with you was formative for me in every way, and this book is only one fraction of everything I learned from you. In particular, I owe so much to the women I have called Sophie, Charlotte, Erin, and Willow—you know who you are and I hope you know how much I appreciate all you have done for me, as well as your continuing friendship. Thanks also to John Mackie for putting into words everything that is beautiful and strange about Spey Bay and for being a wise and true friend.

My constant source of mentorship throughout my academic career has been Sarah Franklin, without whom this book would not have been possible. Your enthusiasm for my tales of Donald Trump, dolphin trivia, and encouragement of my literary idiosyncrasies have fuelled my confidence, whilst your immense insight has kept me from splashing about aimlessly. I must also thank my colleagues at the University of Cambridge, especially Janelle Lamoreaux, for advice, support, and sharing so many of my peculiar preoccupations, and Karen Jent and Zeynep Gurtin for reading various versions and for invaluable editorial suggestions. Thanks to Rhiannon Williams for keeping us all on track and for the wonderful map of Spey Bay.

I am very grateful to Eric Schwartz, my initial editor at Princeton University Press, for all the work he did to secure my contract and to Sarah Caro and Hannah Paul for taking on my project after Eric left for pastures new. I would also like to thank Ali Parrington for taking the book through the production process and Jenn Backer for her thorough copyediting and thoughtful comments. I am especially indebted to the two anonymous reviewers of my manuscript for their excellent advice and constructive criticism.

My research was funded by an ESRC 1+3 studentship, for which I am very grateful. Thanks are also due to my erstwhile colleagues at the LSE, most especially to Fenella Cannell and to my longtime comrade Vicky Boydell. To Rebecca Cassidy and Eric Hirsch, many thanks for your close reading and suggestions. Thanks also to Carrie Heitmeyer, Judith Bovensiepen, Kimberly Chong, Amit Desai, Catherine Allerton, Andrew Sanchez, Indira Arumugam, Ankur Datta, and Liz Frantz for support and friendship along the way. At the University of Edinburgh, where I had an ESRC postdoctoral fellowship before I came to Cambridge, I would especially like to thank Janet Carsten, Jennifer Curtis, Siobhan Magee, and Jennifer Speirs for reading and listening to my accounts of Spey Bay and for helping me stay focused. I must also thank the members of my reading group for their encouragement and support, including most particularly Charlotte Faircloth, Cathy Herbrand, and Jennie Bristow.

Finally, I must thank my family and the non-anthropologist friends who have been there for me throughout. My mother, Juliet Emerson, has always been my biggest fan and my best proofreader. It's impossible to express my gratitude to you. My father, stepmother, brother, and sister have been wonderful and have given me another good reason to visit Scotland regularly. Thanks most especially to Alice Shimmin, Pearlie Kee, Nikki Rummer (who had the misfortune to share a flat with me for much of the time I was writing this), and Barry Watt for keeping the pompoms flying. Thanks to Alana Jelinek for all the discussions about nature we've had in cars, tents, and fields around the country and for laughing at most of my puns.

My partner, Louis Buckley, has given me so much including, not least, the ability to find writing this book easier than I imagined it could be. For your unfailing support, your nest-building abilities, your way with giant vegetables, your sense of fun and your love, thank you so much.

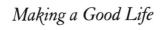

Making a Good Life

The Sperm Whale's Teeth

Early one Friday morning in December 2006 I went with some friends to see the body of a sperm whale that had washed up at Roseisle beach. Roseisle is about a forty-minute drive from the village of Spey Bay, where I lived during fieldwork. This area of Scotland features, amongst other unusual wildlife, a resident population of bottlenose dolphins, and sightings of whales and dolphins are quite common in the area, though to see a sperm whale is rare, as they usually keep to the open seas.

At the beach there were about ten people gathered, including a local journalist. Each person simply looked at the whale, occasionally talking to each other in hushed tones. It lay on its right side in a shallow indentation of sand filled with blood diluted with seawater—a jolting reminder that this had once been a living being. Later, Sophie said she felt an atmosphere of reverence amongst the onlookers. One person touched the dead animal gingerly, as if letting everyone know that she harboured no ill intention; a few others followed as though they had received permission. Despite not having touched the body, Willow said afterwards, "I know it's irrational but I feel sort of unclean, like I need to wash my hands."

The sight of this beached sperm whale was strange and sombre enough, but it soon became clear that this was a more horrific scene than any of us had anticipated. This was the first time I had ever seen a sperm whale in the flesh, but even I knew something was wrong: its lower jaw was missing. Sperm whales, which are the largest of the *odontoceti*, or toothed, whales, are easily recognisable from their boxy, rectangular heads and disproportionately small jaws. I had not realised until this moment that their upper jaw contains no teeth—just a row of depressions into which the large cone-shaped teeth of their narrow lower jaw fit. All that remained where its teeth should have been was a hacked-up stump, dripping fresh blood into the pool below. Tuning into the murmured conversation around me, I heard disgust at this postmortem mutilation on the lips of every person present.

I asked Sophie and Willow, who are actively involved in cetacean conservation and the environmental movement, how they thought this whale had died. They explained that it must have strayed from its natural home in the deep open seas, perhaps disoriented by underwater noise or harassment from boats, searching for its usual diet of squid, whose numbers have declined as a result of contemporary fishing methods. They conjured up an image of a pathetic leviathan eventually giving up the search, its exhausted and starved body washing up on the beach only to suffer the final indignity of having its jaw plundered.

Whether or not they are actively involved in conservation efforts, residents in this region agree that the opportunity to see cetaceans from land and boats in the Moray Firth makes the area special. For the people I knew, this dead whale was a compelling reminder of the potential ecological catastrophes that the world faces. For them, cetaceans represent not only what is good about the natural world but an ethical imperative to conserve and protect it from destructive, unsustainable, and exploitative human activity. By working in cetacean conservation they have placed themselves in the role of carers for these animals and by extension the wider environment. Their ethical labour produces attachments not only to these animals but also to the place and other people. This is salient, as many of them have moved to the area from elsewhere in the UK, brought there by a sense that it is a place that offers a good life. By focusing their efforts on the *local* population of dolphins, they have carved a niche for themselves in the natural and geographical landscape. By focusing particularly on dolphins and whales, rather than the natural world in general, they can also tap into the positive associations that these particular animals have as well as claiming a certain amount of ethical authority for their activities.

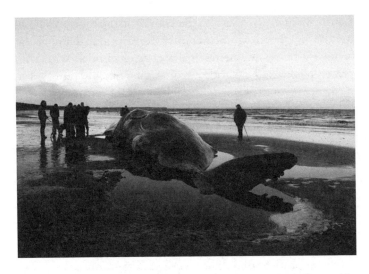

Figure 1. Onlookers at the scene of the stranded sperm whale's body, Roseisle, Moray, December 2006. Photo by author.

Later that day it transpired that the jaw's disappearance was the subject of a criminal investigation. The theft or removal of cetacean body parts is a criminal offence in the UK, not only because many species are legally protected as they are endangered but also because, under the Royal Prerogative, the disposal of beached whales must be approved by the Sovereign, who has an a priori claim to ownership—though the responsibility for dealing with "Royal Fish" (whales measuring twenty-five feet and over) on the Scottish shoreline was devolved to the Scottish Government in 1999.[1]

The police recovered the jaw after a few days, but it was unclear what had happened that December night until I attended a local environmental action group meeting six months later. During a talk, a wildlife crime officer from the local police force indicated that a family from Burghead, a village close to Roseisle, who, as he put it, "act as if they are the local lairds," had taken the jaw. He revealed that it had been recovered after the police offered this family immunity from prosecution in return for its surrender. In the course of their investigation, he told us, they had uncovered three worn-out diamond bit chainsaw blades, numerous pairs of waders filled with congealed blood, and a Landrover that they quickly returned to its owner because of the unbearable stench of rotting flesh that it gave off.

Whatever the motive for this grisly theft, it is clear that the perpetrators were prepared to go to some lengths to acquire these teeth, and the damage to the car it entailed and expensive equipment used suggest that it was not simply for financial gain. National media had reported that local people believe the teeth are "lucky," and during his talk the wildlife crime officer observed that in the Borders region of Scotland, there is a tradition of large families distributing whale teeth amongst their sons to improve fertility. The people I knew dismissed this as an example of the metropolitan press's belief that rural Scotland is a place apart in which, they seem to assume, people are closer to both nature and tradition. They believed instead that the jaw was stolen because the teeth are financially valuable.

The image of well-to-do Scottish landowners circulating wild animal teeth amongst their sons to secure their future generations, like some Caledonian *kula* ring, suggests a close association between kinship, fertility, power, and money. Meanwhile, for the people I lived amongst during fieldwork, the theft signified exploitation of the natural world and the ultimate threat of ecological catastrophe. The teeth therefore represented the ethical imperative for humans to protect and conserve the natural world in order to prevent such destruction. Their sadness at this event was tinged by a sense of failure, all the more poignant given their self-appointed role as guardians of and advocates for the local wildlife and the centrality of this in claiming belonging to the place. Strandings remind us that, whatever similarities we might perceive between humans and cetaceans, the two should not really meet, as when they do, one of them must be out of their element. As we drove back to Spey Bay, Sophie said, "It's so sad to see something so beautiful in life in death. Although it's still beautiful in a way, it's just sad because you get so excited about seeing a sperm whale in the place where you live and then the only opportunity you get is when it's dead."

//

Newspaper reports later confirmed that the whale, an adult male, died from malnutrition.[2] Sperm whales are at the top of the food chain and so it is their unfortunate fate to swallow a lot of the rubbish that ends up in the sea. Necropsies of stranded cetaceans often find plastic bags, probably mistaken for jellyfish, and other such detritus of the contemporary human world inside their stomachs. But, though access to food and a safe environment to live in are of course crucial to survival, the endangerment and extinction of species are ultimately a reproductive failure, the inability to produce future generations.

Whaling was an important industry in Scotland in the eighteenth and nineteenth centuries, and northeastern ports including Aberdeen, Dundee, Peterhead, Fraserburgh, and Banff were the epicentre of Arctic whaling before numbers declined and, later, whaling became morally problematic, then finally illegal. Archaeological evidence suggests that Scots made use of fortuitously (from the human point of view) stranded or caught cetaceans as far back as the Stone Age. They did not eat these whales, but used their bones and teeth as building materials and for making tools and utensils.[3] This was before the many uses of spermaceti[4] had been discovered, which made sperm whales such an attractive target for harpoon-armed commercial whalers later on.

Scientists believe that there is a particularly strong attachment between a sperm whale mother and her calf,[5] though other adult males and females will also care for calves whilst their mothers are feeding.[6] The gestation period for a sperm whale calf is fifteen months and they suckle for at least two years, sometimes communally.[7] As well as spermaceti, another characteristic of sperm whales that made them particularly appealing to whalers was their instinct to herd together and protect their young in the face of danger. As Philip Hoare describes it:

> Threatened sperm whales will stop feeding, swim to the surface, and gather to each other in a cluster. Assembled nose to nose around their calves, they form a tactical circle known as a "marguerite", bodies radiating outwards like the petals of a flower. Thus they present their powerful flukes to any interlopers, protecting their young in a cetacean laager.[8]

This behaviour is thought to be an effective deterrent to orcas, which are the only natural predators that this species face, but it was exploited by whalers, who targeted calves in order to provoke the surrounding pod or herd to gather together, or "heave-to," and protect the young, thus inadvertently providing a ready supply of whales of all ages to harpoon.

Life in a Nature Reserve

Contexts do not neatly condense into symbols;
they must be told through stories that give
them mass and dimension.

—*Rosalind Petchesky*

Reproduction and the Making of Good Lives

What are the environments in which ethics are conceived, lived, and reproduced? This book addresses this question directly by analysing one group of people's ideas about reproduction alongside their everyday ethics. In this ethnography, I explore their ideas about reproduction and assisted reproductive technologies (ART) in a time characterised by the rise of biotechnology, fear of environmental crisis, explicit attention to ethics, and intense public scrutiny of reproduction, parenting, and kinship. My aim is to show that we need to grasp the ways in which reproduction touches on all aspects of life, as well as the ways in which people balance everyday responsibilities and relational commitments with moral values when making ethical judgements.

In public debates about reproduction and particularly ART, the question has tended to be whether a particular decision or technique is ethical or unethical, as if ethics could be reduced to binary moral judgements. This book takes a step back and asks instead, what makes reproduction a matter of ethical attention and concern? Starting with this question allows for a far deeper understanding of what using technology to assist reproduction means, of how it is experienced, and of what effects it has and might have in the future.

This book is based on the ethnographic research I carried out in Spey Bay, a coastal village in northeast Scotland, beginning in late 2005, plus various follow-up trips. My main period of participant observation was twenty months long and included semiformal interviews with nearly thirty of the people I regularly interacted with, which were recorded and transcribed. This ethnography describes the reproductive ethics of a group of middle-class people making "good" lives in Spey Bay who have no personal involvement in ART themselves. As the prologue indicates, these are people who are specifically concerned about the future of the natural world and who see themselves as part of an interconnected and biodiverse environment that is under threat from human activity. As I will show, reproduction and reproductive technologies are enmeshed in larger ethical considerations; for this group of people, these are considerations about how to make a good life and how best to do so in a way that does not harm the environment. By focusing on what people say about reproduction as well as their everyday practices and experiences, I examine how ethics is made through claims and actions, as well as asking what types of knowledge and knowledge practices are at stake in reproductive ethics.

ART have provoked intense public and media debate in the UK as elsewhere, but just whose voices are being heard in these debates? If ART are important, and I think most people would agree that they are, should we only know what they mean to some people? Not only is this a question of getting a fuller picture or more data, it is also questioning a privileged or interested view. It is about taking what "ordinary" people think about these technologies seriously[1] and questioning the way in which public opinion on ART and reproductive ethics has been depicted in the media and in parliament.

As Ann V. Bell's[2] work on inequalities in access to ART amongst people with different socioeconomic statuses in the United States shows, ART are not equally available to all people, and this is true even in the UK despite the fact that the National Health Service (NHS) provides limited infertility treatment to people who meet fairly stringent age and health criteria. Here, ART are largely available to people with a certain amount of money. This is because, in a country that is famously proud of its universal public health care system, most people opt into the private health care system for ART. But it is also because the time spent administering treatments, being tested, and attending doctors' appointments would be difficult for most people to square with the demands of full-time employment and because increasing numbers of people perceive that their best option is to go abroad for fertility treatment. Many people who would like to have children but who have not been able to conceive cannot access technological "fixes"—for medical, economic, and legal reasons—and many believe that even if they did so it would not necessarily remedy their infertility—and, strictly speaking, ART do not treat infertility so much as bypass it.

As Sarah Franklin has shown, in the UK IVF is a "platform technology," providing the basis for research and development into stem cell therapies, regenerative medicine, and genetic testing. The British government also sees it as fertile ground for developing the lucrative biotechnology industry. As she puts it, "A long legacy of public support for increasingly radical forms of human embryo research, combined with explicit cross-party support for ongoing innovation in this field, has embedded a logic that is now seemingly part of the British national imaginary, and is celebrated as a source of national pride."[3] If we consider this bigger picture, it seems that, in fact, there are very few people who are not affected by ART in the UK. It also hints at some of the specific interests that are influencing public debates about ART.

An important observation that has arisen from a number of clinic-based ethnographies is that ART can place greater pressure on infertile people to try, or to be seen to be trying, every possible remedy for their childlessness.[4] As well as putting specific pressures on particular individuals and couples, these technologies have probably contributed to a trend towards greater medicalisation of reproduction and infertility, as well as a sense that the decision not to have children, whether or not one is infertile, is an aberrant or pathetic one. It may also be that the availability of ART has contributed to a parenting culture that puts pressure on parents to maximise every opportunity to improve the health and future of their children or risk being stigmatised and even prosecuted as a "bad" parent. In other words, we are all implicated in ART.

ART do, of course, bring joy and relief to many people, and my intention is certainly not to belittle the anguish that infertility causes many people, to recommend that they should not have access to medical assistance to help them conceive, or to imply that individuals who are infertile—or, for that matter, gay or single parents—should shoulder the responsibility for wider social, legal, economic, or political inequalities. Instead, I simply want to keep sight of the fact that, as many of the early feminist critics of ART pointed out,[5] reproductive technologies are not politically or ethically neutral. As many of these scholars predicted, despite their apparently revolutionary and radical potential, they can be critical in the protection, reproduction, and promotion of established norms and ideologies of kinship, sexuality, and gender. As the continuing and lucrative normalisation and development of these technologies show, it is not only social norms that are being protected by ART but also the industry that creates, develops, and "translates" them into financial returns.[6] It seems a little strange, given this, that we know so little about what "ordinary" people—that is, not patients, clinicians, medical researchers, politicians, bioethicists, or theologians, but *everyone else*—think about these technologies, when they are the context that provides the ground for and also receives the effects, positive and negative, radical and conservative, that these technologies bring about.

Technologies are made by people in particular contexts, they are developed by people in particular contexts, and they are used by people in particular contexts. In his classic study of another defining technology of the twentieth century, television, Raymond Williams pointed out the dangers of attributing agency to technologies,[7] such as in the idea that violent films cause higher homicide rates. He counsels us to question the assumption that television or any other technology can cause any particular social effect and warns against the idea that technologies originate in isolation. Williams charts how television developed in a context in which it made sense and seemed to meet certain needs, from the desire of people to communicate across distances in a period of greater geographical mobility, to the centralisation of political power, to the development of the mass media. However, in assessing the causes and effects of technologies, he says, we must be careful not to throw the baby out with the bathwater:

> While we have to reject technological determinism, in all its forms, we must be careful not to substitute for it the notion of a determined technology. . . . Determination is a real social process, but never (as in some theological and some Marxist versions) a wholly controlling, wholly predicting set of causes. On the contrary, the reality of determination is the setting of limits and the exertion of pressures, within which variable social practices are profoundly affected but never necessarily controlled. We have to think of determination not as a single force, or a single abstraction of forces, but as a process in which real determining factors—the distribution of power or of capital, social and physical inheritance, relations of scale and size between groups—set limits and exert pressures, but neither wholly control nor wholly predict the outcome of complex activity within or at these limits, and under or against these pressures.[8]

One of the major arguments of this book is that we need, as researchers, citizens, or activists, to attend to the importance of what reproduction and ART mean to whole communities and not only to individuals who are consumers, or purveyors, of these technologies. The fact that ART have been so hotly and publicly contested in the UK and elsewhere indicates that reproduction and ART affect all our lives—not only in our own individual reproductive decision making but because questions about how, when, if, and with whom (if anyone) we have children seem to reflect something about who we are as a community or society. We should be asking what our ideas about reproduction and ART tell us about ourselves. The good news is that social scientific research methods provide us with the tools to do that, as this book will show.

Reproduction, Bioethics, and Context

The ethical questions that reproduction and reproductive technologies seem to inevitably raise have been exercising politicians, theologians, feminists, and others for many decades now. Alongside this, there has been a continuous interest in the same sorts of questions amongst social scientists. As their work reminds us, reproduction provokes different kinds of ethical questions and relates to different conceptions of ethics. Thus debates about the ethics of abortion, for example, may be, amongst other things, about limiting or extending legal rights to certain forms of life, the morality of denying medical services to the poor, medical ethics, the ontological status of embryos and foetuses, exposing coercive sexual encounters, upholding religious doctrine, recognising gender inequalities in child care and work, protecting particular populations through pro-natalist policies or preventing reproduction amongst certain groups according to eugenicist ideologies, assumptions about the nature of bodily autonomy, or the desirability of medical interventions in human reproduction. Whilst each of these considerations might be broken down into different domains—law, politics, civil rights, professional conduct, and so on—they are also each in their own way ethical questions, as they demand that people reflect on what is the good thing to do, or the best reason to take one course of action and not another. When making public claims intended to effect political, social, or legal change, advocates of certain positions will often select particular strands and pull on them to weave together their arguments. Seeking to pull apart these different types of ethical questions rather than working within their interconnectedness may, then, be an interested move with particular aims.

The major academic discipline to focus its attention on ART, in addition to scholars in sociology, anthropology, and science and technology studies, has been bioethics. Since its inception, bioethics has been closely associated with questions about reproduction, initially focusing on abortion but increasingly on ART and associated techniques. Alongside questions about the beginning and end of life and the informed consent of patients and participants in medical research, a major consideration that has exercised bioethics is the issue of payment or compensation for bodily "products" and "services." Melinda Cooper and Catherine Waldby have recently argued that "bioethics as discourse and practice is internal to the political economy of the life sciences,"[9] even when it takes a principled position against bodily commodification. So, in a post-Fordist world of precarious, transnational, and informal labour, the bioethical principle of compensation rather than payment can propel large numbers of people into acting as vendors of tissues and as research subjects in order to supplement low incomes and to access health care for themselves. The valorisation of informed consent, they argue, contributes to this as egg vendors, surrogate mothers, and embryo donors are effectively signing away their right to seek redress for any harm caused by participating in the fertility industry or clinical research, thus exposing themselves not only to the bodily risks of such procedures but also the risks of precarious and informal "work."

In the UK, bioethicists are more familiar figures in public debates about reproductive technologies than are social scientists, and they also provide advice to government and regulators. Bioethics is both a response to medical technologies that create, extend, and end life and a by-product of them. The development of this discipline not only reflects a burgeoning of technologies that seem to challenge ethical assumptions and modes of medical practice but also implies a consensus that bioethical questions are important and complex enough to warrant the development of specialist expertise beyond the clinic or lab. As I will argue here,[10] it is important to remember the contexts into which both bioethics and ART were born, as well as to question just what makes any particular treatment or technology a subject of bioethical concern.

Historically, the dialogue between bioethicists and social scientists has centred on questions of universalism versus particularism, which generally speaking reflects a broad disciplinary difference in that bioethicists seek to identify and even prescribe ethical practice whilst social scientists aim to describe and understand it. One important example of this is a special issue of the academic journal *Daedalus* titled "Bioethics and Beyond" edited by Arthur Kleinman, Renée C. Fox, and Arthur M. Brandt and published in 1999. In this issue, Kleinman articulates the importance of social scientific insights to bioethics:

> Bioethics is confronted with an extraordinarily difficult quandary: how to reconcile the clearly immense differences in the social and personal realities of moral life with the need to apply a universal standard to those fragments of experience that can foster not only comparison and evaluation but also action. For philosophers, the gulf between the universal and the particular may be regarded as an irksome and perennial barrier; but bioethicists, like clinicians and policy implementers, simply cannot function without finding a way of relating ethical deliberation to local contexts.[11]

One particularly important point that Kleinman makes is that the critique of universalism in bioethics that many social scientists have made is not an attempt to undermine a competing discipline but to suggest that if bioethicists were to attend to some of the findings of social scientific research, this could inform, and therefore strengthen, bioethical analysis, policy, and practice[12]—and, by implication, make it more ethical. As

Kleinman suggests and leading American bioethicist Daniel Callahan[13] confirms, there is an intractable tension between social scientists' and bioethicists' approaches to ethics because the latter are—albeit to varying degrees and with different sympathies—committed to finding widely, if not universally, applicable principles. But that does not mean that the other side of the coin is social scientists dogmatically promoting cultural relativism. It is instead about problematising a discipline that can, in its insistence on generalisable principles, succumb to paternalism and even moral imperialism.[14]

Another important point that comes out of this debate is the individualism inherent in bioethics and the difficulty it has had with conceiving of ethics in a way that accounts for more communitarian values and experiences, which in my view reflects a stereotypical picture of people in Western countries as being primarily self-interested. This debate also points to a division between ethics as a constant process of self-fashioning and lived practice on the one hand and ethics as a set of codified principles governing a particular profession or practice on the other. Bioethics, by its very nature, is required to prioritise principles over practices, which can mean failing to fully recognise the fact that professional ethics and the wider ethical values and practices of the societies in which doctors and researchers operate are inseparable.

Like Kleinman, Barry Hoffmaster[15] has argued for bioethics' greater engagement with social scientific research, based on his sense that bioethics should be as much about understanding ethical decisions as justifying them. Hoffmaster believes that a bioethics that is "situated in lived human experience,"[16] informed by social scientists' findings, is a better bioethics. He also draws attention to the importance of emotions in ethical decisions:

> Putting bioethics in personal, social, and cultural contexts opens the way for modes of moral deliberation that are not general, rational, and impartial but that embrace the distinctive histories, relationships, and milieus of people and engage

their emotions as much as their reason. Such a bioethics also recognizes the multiple backgrounds—institutional, economic, historical, and political—that structure moral problems and give meanings to moral concepts. This is a bioethics situated in lived human experience. The qualitative research approaches of the social sciences, ethnography in particular, can be used to explore the moral dimensions of that experience and thus to enhance our understanding of the nature of morality and its place in our lives. The ultimate goal of this endeavor is a bioethics that is more attuned to the particular and more sensitive to the personal—a bioethics that is more humane and more helpful.[17]

Of course, in order to convince bioethicists that they need to incorporate social scientific research into their work they will have to be persuaded of the importance of context in ethical decision making, and it seems that there is still work to do in this respect. Bioethicists, along with policymakers and regulators, need to understand that context is not a euphemism for mitigating circumstances but instead a way of attuning oneself to the contingent realities of people's lives. Nonetheless, bioethics has taken "an empirical turn,"[18] with direction from some of the leading figures in bioethics, including Daniel Callahan, cofounder of the Hastings Center, for greater attention to alternative moral positions within bioethics. I would sound a note of caution here. Both bioethicists and social scientists should remember that questions of universals and particulars are not the same as questions of Western and non-Western values. That is, whilst bioethicists should certainly attend to other moral worlds and try to develop models that take account of the multiple interests that may be at stake in any particular ethical decision, they should not assume that we know Western moralities by reading them off from laws or professional codes of conduct or that moral philosophy is a mirror onto "Western ethics."

Bioethics is itself shaped by its context, just as the social sciences are, but we cannot assume that that context is simply

something that can be labelled "Western culture." As Duncan
Wilson says about the development of bioethics in the UK, "the
'bioethical' aspects of particular practices and objects were not
self-evident, but were the product of specific socio-political contexts and professional agendas in the late twentieth century."
He therefore urges us to consider what made certain treatments
and technologies worthy of the attention of bioethicists (and, by
extension, what made others unworthy of such attention).[19] In
Britain, Wilson writes, bioethics did not have much sway until
the 1980s. Similarly, and probably not coincidentally, the birth
of the first IVF baby, Louise Brown, in 1978 and the initial expansion of IVF were largely viewed positively, but by the 1980s,
there were increasing calls for greater external oversight of doctors and researchers in the media, and lawyers and philosophers
started to enter the public debate, which dovetailed with the
new Conservative government's desire to see greater "accountability" amongst professions and the promotion of (consumer)
choice in all aspects of life.[20] A further important point that
Wilson makes is that, though some bioethicists have asserted
that the discipline has its roots in the civil rights movement and
a left-wing concern with medical paternalism, bioethics in the
UK only took off because the call for greater oversight resonated
with the Thatcherite political climate of the 1980s and because
bioethicists portrayed themselves to the medical profession as
helpers at least as much as critics.[21]

In the British and Scottish parliaments, debates about reproduction, including abortion, ART, and, most recently, treatments for mitochondrial disease, are treated as "matters of conscience," so politicians deciding how to regulate them do so off
their own bat rather than according to the party line, which
already hints at some of the complexities of reproductive ethics, even in the soundbite-friendly world of political wrangling.
The fact that differing moral positions are conventionally respected in this way also implies a tacit assumption that there
are no universal right answers with which to settle such ethical
questions.

What I want to suggest here is that there is something else missing from our picture of public debates about ART, and that is the ethics of people who are not using these technologies themselves but who are concerned about them and about what they mean, who have rarely been the subject of research. This is partly a problem of representation and a reflection of the fact that both politics and the media favour succinct and generalisable data over the complex and nuanced accounts that qualitative sociologists and anthropologists (and, I'm sure, some bioethicists) deal in, but I think it also suggests a sense that medical technologies only affect those who are treated with them, which is untenable. One clear empirical point that this book illustrates is that it is very difficult to untangle reproduction from people's everyday concerns, and this is not only true for the infertile.

By describing and analysing what people in Spey Bay think about the ethics of reproduction and ART, this book questions whether public commentators, journalists, and politicians have grasped the complexity and thoughtfulness of the responses to these technologies of people who have no personal involvement in them—and why they are important. Charis Thompson has discussed the "public domain of bioethics" in her study of ART in the United States. She writes,

> The British have a habit of putting prominent individuals from various domains—members of the proverbial "Great and the Good"—on committees that produce recommendations about matters of public concern that can lead to regulatory capacity. And in Britain, it is still possible for a single prominent expert in the field to become an honored and well-known public spokesperson.[22]

Thompson contrasts this with the American context, where she says that whilst "in some sense . . . the public is saturated with reproductive technologies," through fictional and popular depictions of them in soap operas, novels, and magazine articles (which could also be said of the UK), "conspicuously missing is anything approaching an agora of ideas where the public can openly and equally discuss the pros and cons of reproductive technologies. Indeed, it is hard even to imagine what the space, the technologies of dissemination, mitigation, and aggregation, and the rhetorics of this agora might be."[23] She then goes on to analyse the importance of various iterations of the ethic of privacy in maintaining this absence of agora in the American context.

Thompson's point about privacy and her implication that relying on those affected by infertility to be pioneers of the technologies' development will probably lead to greater stratification is very important. I would only add that I am unsure how successful attempts to create such a public domain in the UK have been as well. The problem is that public discussions of reproductive ethics have been more about setting moral prescriptions and legal proscriptions than reflecting people's rich ethical deliberations. I would suggest that the agora is ill equipped for understanding reproductive ethics, as it has little interest in recognising the contingent and processual nature of ethics or in knowing the contexts in which we make ethics from the bottom up. This is a problem for how we think about ART now and in the future, and it is one that this book speaks to directly.

In this book, I depart from the bioethical approach to reproduction and ART by emphasising the contingent and contextual nature of ethics and by working from the assumption that, in everyday life and in reproduction, ethics is constantly made. I am much less interested in trying to provide a definitive account of people in Spey Bay's reproductive ethics than in following the making of their ethical judgements and how these connect with their everyday ethical values and priorities.[24] The approach I am taking, led by my data, is more akin to an ethics of care approach, which, as Annemarie Mol and colleagues have noted, is different from that of medical ethics or bioethics, in that it "never sought to answer what is good, let alone to do so from the outside."[25] This is an approach that recognises that in people's everyday lives, ethics is not so much about abstract moral reasoning but about taking other perspectives into account and considering how any decision affects all those involved.[26] It is a way of looking at the world through interrelation and connection rather than in neat divisions.

Thanks for All the Fish

This ethnography is unusual not only in that it relates the ethical views of people who have no personal involvement in ART but also in that this is a group of people who are used to thinking and talking about ethics, nature, humanity, and the future as they go about their everyday lives. Whilst focused on a small and particular group of people, this book carries questions of how humans should reproduce themselves onto a much wider terrain than does existing work on reproductive ethics and ART. People in Spey Bay think about nature and the limits of the natural on a quotidian basis and this is, as I hope to show through this ethnography, fertile ground for thinking about reproduction and how it connects with other aspects of life. In the remainder of this chapter, I will introduce the context for this project, by starting to describe Spey Bay, the people who work and live there, and their everyday concerns, before ending with an outline of the book's structure.

Spey Bay is a tiny village in the county of Moray (pronounced: *Murrie*) in northeast Scotland. It is perched at the mouth of the River Spey on the picturesque Moray Firth coast, a place at times windy and spindrift-flecked, at others a tranquil, sunny haven. Here the Spey's peat-browned freshwater, filtered through the Cairngorm Mountains, reaches the end of its long journey in a cataclysmic encounter with the chilly saltwater of the North Sea. Being at the confluence of a powerful river and a churning sea, the sand and shingle banks of the bay are in constant flux, with the river's force constantly hewing fresh margins to its passage.

The village of Spey Bay lies within a 450-hectare nature reserve, beside the Speyside Way long-distance footpath. Spey Bay

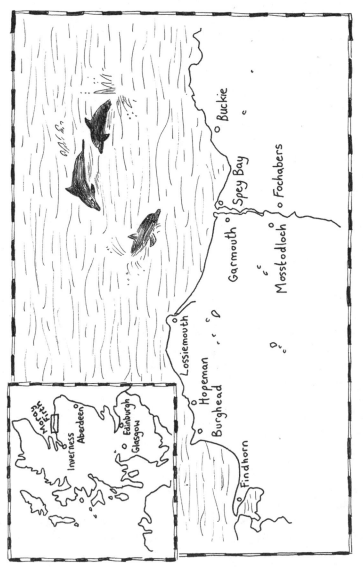

Figure 2. Map of Spey Bay and the surrounding area. Illustration by Rhiannon Williams.

is designated a Site of Special Scientific Interest (SSSI), and the Inner Moray Firth is a Special Area of Conservation because of its population of bottlenose dolphins, which are thought of as vulnerable[27] as they are a small group and because they reproduce slowly,[28] and a Wetland of International Importance because it is a breeding ground for various rare birds including osprey, which were once extinct in the UK. The Spey is also home to a population of Atlantic salmon, which provided the original reason for the area's settlement. Drawn close to the coast by the salmon, trout, and other fish in the river, dolphins and whales are regularly spotted along the firth, especially during the spring and summer. The human inhabitants of the villages along the coast associate themselves with dolphins on village name signs and in the decor and products of local businesses. Moray's scenic coastline, rare wildlife, and dramatic landscape all contribute to a common sense that it is an altogether more natural place offering a better way of life. This implies a critical contrast with other parts of the country, typically more suggestive than literal, but that plays into long-established rhetorical rivalries between the country and the city in British culture.[29]

Spey Bay is tucked away from other settlements, usually approached by a winding five-mile road alongside the Spey from Fochabers (see Figure 2). During my time living there, I became familiar with the sense of being enclosed by a ring of warmth and intimacy and the shift of perspective onto the small scale of my immediate surroundings once in Spey Bay. The road to Spey Bay marks both a phenomenological and spatial boundary. Inside, I felt part of something—something different and, implicitly, better. Many times whilst I was walking along the beach, collecting logs for the fire or feeding Sophie's chickens, a passing visitor would remark on how lucky I was to live there.

The immediate presence of the sea once you arrive in Spey Bay also makes it feel like a frontier. Coastal Moray is roughly bi-seasonal, seeming to come alive in the spring and summer, when migrating birds start to return, dolphin sightings begin, and the first wave of tourists visit, whilst during the long autumn and winter it closes in on itself and your willingness to stay through the cold, dark nights is testament to your status as a resident rather than a visitor. The daily weather in this corner of the world is changeable and highly localised. One week in Spey Bay in late March 2007, for example, opened with gale-force winds, horizontal snow, and extremely rough seas, but a few days later I was eating lunch outside in mild sunshine. Locals know how to manage themselves in the climate and can find beauty in a boiling sea or a fog-bound beach.

In contrast to the Highlands that border it, which are visible across the firth on fine days, Moray enjoys fertile and productive land and great swathes of the area are set aside for agriculture; this is particularly evident in the low-lying area of coastal Moray from Fochabers to Brodie called the Laich[30] of Moray. The palette of the place is more varied than the browns, greens, and purples of the Highlands, with bright yellow broom and coconut-scented gorse visible for much of the year, the ever-changing silver-grey-blue swirl of the sea, the pink pebbles and yellow-peach sands of the beaches, and the primary colours of the fishing boats in the harbours. People frequently referred to Spey Bay and Moray as places of natural beauty. When they did so, they were referring to emotion and embodied experience as much as aesthetic appreciation. A beautiful landscape in this case conjures up images of being outdoors, looking out to sea, feeling the wind and sun on your face, contemplating the distant hills, and appreciating the flora and fauna, which goes along with the sense that this is a place where people have more time to appreciate their surroundings, whether that be land, animals, plants, or other people. People here feel that they live closer to the natural world, an idea that is not only deeply fulfilling since, as we shall see, they value nature so highly, but also promotes action, since there is a sense that having all this on your doorstep makes the imperative to care for the environment all the more pressing. Living in a naturally beautiful place is a responsibility.

Spey Bay was built on salmon fishing and golf. Tugnet, at one end of Spey Bay, was, as the name indicates, the base for a large fish-processing operation in the nineteenth and twentieth centuries. Salmon fishing at Tugnet started in the twelfth century, with people fishing on the river from handmade coracles as well as from the shore. In the sixteenth century, the land-owner the Duke of Gordon expanded the fishing operation to supply the English market. By then, men fished from slightly larger boats called cobles. There has never been a harbour at Spey Bay, but a salmon fishing station with accommodation for the staff was built in 1768 and the buildings still stand today. It employed one hundred and fifty people at its peak.

In the eighteenth century the industry turned to transporting fresh salmon packed in ice, and an icehouse, reputed to be the largest in Scotland, was built in Tugnet in 1791 and expanded in 1830. It was used to store the ice, cut from the river in winter, in which the fish were packed before being sent south to London on the railway which ran along the Moray Firth coast and stopped just south of Spey Bay itself. Although salmon is not fished on an industrial scale on the Spey anymore and the train line has long been out of commission, the deep-sea fishing industry is still active along the coastline of Moray and Aberdeenshire, though it has changed much in recent decades.[31] Unfortunately I did not come into contact with those who worked in fishing except for the occasional encounter with retired fishermen visiting Spey Bay, who sometimes remarked with wistful authority upon the number of times they had seen dolphins and whales bow-riding whilst out fishing, but Jane Nadel-Klein has written about the local fishing communities here.[32]

The Tugnet salmon fishing operation closed in the 1990s, but this same complex of ashlar buildings is still the home of the largest employer in the village and one of the most popular tourist attractions in northeast Scotland, a wildlife centre that was opened by a local couple in 1997 and is now run by an international cetacean conservation charity. I learned much of the history of Tugnet fishing from staff at the wildlife centre, who tell it to visitors as they take them on tours around the icehouse. The wildlife centre operates on a nonprofit basis and is staffed by a handful of paid employees plus volunteers. The contrasts between fishing and cetacean conservation suggest much about the way that employment and industry have changed in this village and in the wider area, as the Moray Firth coast has gradually shifted from being focused on the fishing industry to becoming associated with leisure and tourism, which reflects a wider decline in manufacturing and an increase in tourism in the national economy of Scotland. One survey from 2009 found that the financial value of whale- and dolphin-watching tourism in the Moray Firth area is over £10 million.[33] Other surveys show that there is generally a favourable attitude towards cetaceans and their conservation in Scotland: 80 percent of Scots surveyed supported the idea of introducing a specific law to protect cetaceans and 40 percent agreed that if a politician proposed such a law they would see her or him in a more favourable light.[34]

The Save the Whale campaign was one of the first and in many ways defining moments in the history of the twentieth-century Green movement.[35] The state of whales and dolphins is treated as metonymic of the environment and cetaceans continue to be one of the most popular conservation causes. One reason for the success of this particular cause is the fact that dolphins and whales are "charismatic megafauna" and popularly thought of as benign (or even altruistic), intelligent, social, and family oriented. In the Moray Firth area, the local population of over one hundred bottlenose dolphins are metonymic not only of the place but of people's ethical, political, and social values. Just as Rebecca Cassidy[36] showed in her exemplary study of horseracing society in Newmarket, this kinship between people and dolphins in Spey Bay is a manifestation of the fact that Western people can in fact reach across the human-animal divide. In Spey Bay this kinship is with wild animals rather than domesticated ones, but dolphins and whales also provoke people to reconsider their own place in, and relationship to, nature.

Whales and dolphins are very important in the identity of people in this area, but their meanings have certainly shifted over the centuries. During my fieldwork, I had assumed that this friendly association between people and cetaceans was a relatively recent phenomenon that had emerged alongside the decline in North Sea fishing and the mainstreaming of concerns about the environment. Certainly these factors are important to contemporary ideas about cetaceans and especially to their ethical value. However, this interest does seem to have historical precedents. Marine biologist E.C.M. Parsons has argued that the number of carvings of "Pictish beasts," which appear to be cetaceans, and probably dolphins, on standing stones in northeast Scotland indicates that cetaceans have been culturally significant in Scotland since the Iron Age.[37] Parsons suggests that Saint Columba's encounter with a strange creature that later became thought of as the Loch Ness Monster (or, more likely, one of its antecedents) may in fact have been a whale in the Moray Firth. He also says that the unicorn that features on Scotland's Royal Crest is likely to be inspired by sightings of narwhals that could have ranged as far as the waters around Scotland in the chilly climate of the Middle Ages and Renaissance.[38] Though I am a little sceptical about gauging cultural meanings from such slight evidence, I must admit that these examples are appealing. Whatever the historical veracity of these claims, the efforts some contemporary researchers have gone to in order to find links between humans and cetaceans in Scotland does at the very least reinforce the deep significance that these animals have today.

Making a Home

The former Tugnet fishing station is a square courtyard of one- and two-storey buildings, just a few metres from the Spey mouth to its west and the sea to the north. The former station manager's house flanks the courtyard entrance (see Figure 3) and looks not to the sea but south along the Spey to Ben Rinnes, whose 841 metres I once climbed with some of my friends from Spey Bay shod, despite the snow, in nothing more specialist than wellington boots. The house has now been split in two and Sophie,[39] the wildlife centre manager, rented the smaller of these houses and the charity that runs the wildlife centre rented the house next door as accommodation for the residential volunteers. When I moved to Spey Bay I lived in the volunteer accommodation for around six months and then moved in with Sophie next door after her housemate Steve bought a flat in the nearest city, Elgin. Two families live in the two other houses in the courtyard. Next to the volunteers' accommodation is the wildlife centre office and, beyond that, the centre, wildlife garden, and café. The buildings are owned and let by The Crown Estate.[40]

Apart from the wildlife centre, the only other public facility in Spey Bay itself is the village hall, which is the venue for community events and leisure activities such as quiz nights, ceilidhs, and yoga classes. People sometimes voiced disappointment that there is no pub in the village, and thus no social focal point. There is a hotel, but during my fieldwork it was closed, though golfers could use its course. The nearest pub and food shop are in Garmouth, on the other bank of the Spey. However, they are only nearest as the crow flies or if you are walking—by road, the closest amenities are in Fochabers, five miles inland. Fochabers, with a population of around two thousand, is home to the Baxter's food manufacturing business and also has a primary school and high school, doctor's surgery, veterinary practice, pubs, grocery stores, two butchers, a fish and chip shop, a handful of other independent shops, and two churches.

Throughout this ethnography, I use "people in Spey Bay" as a shorthand for all those I met, spoke to, and got to know during fieldwork, whether or not they actually lived in the village of Spey Bay and whether or not we were actually in Spey Bay at the time of each particular event or conversation recounted. Whilst this shorthand relies on a little literary license, it does reflect the fact that Spey Bay is where I was based for fieldwork and that I met most people there or through other people I had met there. It also captures the way in which Spey Bay and the work of the wildlife centre there epitomise the ethical values that inform how people make good lives here. Throughout the book, I will

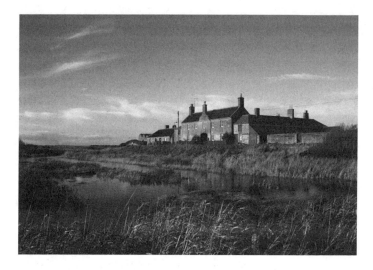

Figure 3. Tugnet viewed from the Speyside Way, looking northwest. The main building in the centre of the picture is the former fishing station manager's house, in which I lived during fieldwork. The single-storey building to its left is the back entrance to the wildlife centre, and to the left of that, with the three humps on the roof, is the icehouse. The Spey mouth lies just beyond the icehouse and the beach is on the other side of the buildings. Photo by author.

mention where particular individuals live and where they come from in order to try to remind the reader that this is not an isolated community of people born and bred in Spey Bay.

Sophie was the social lynchpin of the group of people I met during fieldwork. She grew up in rural northwestern England and went to university in Scotland. She spent the years in between graduating and moving to Spey Bay working in various charities in the UK and abroad. She enjoys hiking, cycling, wildlife-watching, and other outdoor pursuits but also modern art, world music, and foreign cuisine. Sophie had lived in Spey Bay for four years when I first met her and was never short of superlatives to describe the place. When I asked her if she felt that Spey Bay was her home she agreed emphatically, adding that what was important was that she *felt at home* there.

Sophie is an extremely warm, enthusiastic person who devotes most of her time and energy to doing things for other people, and she was notorious for her tendency to spontaneously invite people to dinner or to stay at her house, which I quickly became accustomed to after I moved in with her myself. One of my foremost mental images of Spey Bay is her orange sherbet–coloured sitting room with its flickering open fire, Indian throws for curtains, disco ball, multicoloured rug, large and well-used dining table, huge stacks of CDs, and hookah pipe in one corner. On the walls were a poster of a turtle, a memento of a Caribbean conservation project she had worked on, a framed photograph of the north Highlands where she spent family holidays as a child, a world map annotated by hand with notes of her and her friends' travels, and a felt painting of a tern made by a friend and former colleague who had settled in the area after falling in love with a local man.

The colleagues and friends who worked in the wildlife centre would often eat together in each other's houses after work or on the weekends. These were usually short-notice, informal gatherings, and both Sophie's house and the volunteers' accommodation next door had something of a tacit open-door policy, with a steady flow of people dropping in through the day. At these shared meals, food came from mixed sources including supermarkets, organic veg-boxes,[41] the local butcher, and people's own gardens. People would make a variety of dishes to cater to the differing tastes and dietary requirements of guests, and typically individuals would contribute different dishes or bring drinks to spread cost and labour. The efforts that went into these meals are exemplary of the ethic of care that people in Spey Bay enact in their daily interactions with each other, whilst the complicated choreography of sourcing these meals offers a microcosmic view of living in a consumer society whilst also attempting to resist some of those values.

Friends in Spey Bay are expected to be closely involved in each other's lives and to share confidences, and this is facilitated by the routine proximity in which they live and work. Spey Bay is a very sociable place. As well as the steady stream of shared meals, there were regular parties and people would get together for day trips, walks, and even visits to the supermarket (which also saved on petrol). Friends were informal with each other in a way that is reminiscent of kin; teasing and joking were an important part of social life and reflect their close intimacy. Inevitably the other side to this is gossip, and people did occasionally complain about information that they had told others in confidence somehow finding its way into public circulation. Trusting outsiders or newcomers with sensitive information was also a means of testing the boundaries of the group. If people could accept the more negative aspects of life in such a close-knit community, with few secrets and a limited range of cultural activities, that suggested that they could fit in there. Individuals were conceptualised as living in overlapping networks of reciprocity and mutual support and were encouraged to "be themselves," however eccentric or singular that self may be. Of course, certain differences were less likely to be tolerated, such as climate change scepticism, but differences in ethnic origin, sexual orientation, age, or socioeconomic background were generally accepted as part of life and, indeed, what make people "interesting."[42]

Despite this self-conscious embracing of diversity, the people I met during fieldwork are a very homogenous group. Though staff and volunteers in the wildlife centre come from across the UK, Western Europe, and North America, almost all were white and middle class. A handful had been in single-sex relationships and/or did not identify as heterosexual, though as I will note in later chapters, when I talked with those who did not have children about their plans for future parenthood they assumed that they would have children within a heterosexual relationship. One unusual feature of this group, given that one of the things they have in common is their work, is that women are in the majority. As I will discuss further in the next chapter, the vast majority of the paid staff and most of the residential volunteers[43] at the wildlife centre were women, though the local volunteers, who help out on a less frequent basis, were more evenly split in gender. Most of the paid staff and residential volunteers were in their mid-twenties to mid-thirties, whilst the local volunteers were either similar ages or in their fifties to sixties.

As this is an ethnographic study, I did not seek a representative sample and in many ways the strength of this particular case is its specificity. It is worth briefly noting the demographic profile of the area, though, to give a broader sense of this region. The following figures are taken from the most recent census, in 2011.[44] Whilst in terms of age, marriage, and gender statistics Moray's profile is very similar to the picture for Scotland as a whole, it is quite different in terms of the ethnicity and nationality of residents. So, whilst 4 percent of the population in Scotland are Asian or Black, in Moray just over 1 percent are. Notably, the number of white migrants in Moray is also lower than for Scotland as a whole. Given these figures, it is perhaps unsurprising that there is such little ethnic diversity amongst people working in the wildlife centre. At the centre, Scottish people were in the minority and only one person had grown up in Moray. The most recent census shows that in Moray, just under 78 percent are "White—Scottish," whilst 18 percent are "White—other British." For Scotland as a whole, by comparison, 84 percent are "White—Scottish" and just under 8 percent are "White—other British." A major reason for this preponderance of non-Scottish Britons in the county is the presence of Royal Air Force (RAF) personnel and their families at RAF Lossiemouth and RAF Kinloss (the latter of which has since become an army barracks). A handful of staff and volunteers in the wildlife centre were the female partners of men who work in the RAF, but Moray is also known as a place that people from elsewhere in the UK retire to.

The perception that living in the countryside is beneficial to people's well-being is a longstanding one in the UK, and moving to a more rural location with a "slower" pace of life and beautiful landscape is a common aspiration, though it is of course one that appeals most to people who feel comfortable in the countryside and is only accessible to people who can find work there or have independent means. Survey figures from around the time that I was in Moray found that half of British people living in urban areas wanted to move to the country, whilst only one in ten rural residents would prefer to live elsewhere.[45] In his study of English migrants to Scotland, Murray Watson analysed participants' multilayered reasons for moving.[46] Many of these resonate with those of people here, suggesting that their motives for seeking a good life in Spey Bay overlap with popular perceptions of what life in Scotland is like. In particular, many of his respondents identified Scotland as a place where you can get away from the fast pace and pressures of urban British life to enjoy a better way of living[47] and cited the landscape and scenery of Scotland as a motivating factor in their migrations.[48]

In terms of understanding the context in which I did this research, it is important to remember that my main period of fieldwork ended shortly before the global financial crisis took hold. At the time, there were rumours of a "credit crunch," but it was still another year before Lehman Brothers went into administration and the bailout of Royal Bank of Scotland Group PLC and other banks in the UK. The crisis of the time seemed not so much financial as political, or existential, with the War on Terror looming large in the collective psyche. The 7/7 attacks on the London public transport system happened in 2005, whilst I was preparing to start my fieldwork, and car bomb plots targeting two sites in London and Glasgow International Airport were foiled in June 2007, not long before I returned to London. Though no one told me that they had moved to Spey Bay to get away from the risk of terrorist attacks, they did feel that it was safer in the countryside[49] than in cities, and in my field notes in the days following the foiled attempt to bomb Glasgow airport I noted how relieved I was to be in a place that was highly unlikely ever to be targeted by terrorists.

The decision to move to Moray for the people I met there was primarily a positive choice towards achieving certain goals rather than away from an unpleasant past. This goes along with their more general orientation towards the future rather than the past, which contrasts with many other British communities that have been described by ethnographers. For instance, in *Born and Bred*, Jeanette Edwards describes Bacup, Lancashire, as a place in which the present is scarred by memories and imaginings of its industrial past, manifested in both nostalgia and anxiety about the future.[50] She also shows that in many ways community is celebrated and sought there because people feel they have lost it. The idea of community can, then, often refer to a sense of endangerment, and in chapter 2 I will discuss the salience of environmentalist ideas about endangerment to reproduction and the future in Spey Bay. In Spey Bay, people's ideas about community and relationships with others are influenced not by a sense of loss,[51] a desire to recapture something from their past,[52] or indeed a straightforward rejection of prevailing mores but instead part of a process of coming to belong somewhere and building connections to others in a place in which they quickly come to feel at home. In this case, community is more about conserving the conditions for a good future than re-creating a past idyll.

Internal migration within Britain is not especially unusual, particularly amongst middle-class people, who frequently move around to study and work. Though most people in Spey Bay have good relationships with their parents and siblings, the fact that many of them have moved away from their families demonstrates that their vision of a good life does not necessarily include living close to them, especially when there are supportive and like-minded friends on hand. One obvious drawback of being away from families for younger people is that their practical and material support is harder to access, including for example if they later come to have children themselves, though this did not seem to concern many of the people I knew, as they were currently more interested in finding personal fulfilment through their work and interests, although some single women did express minor concerns about their chances of meeting a future partner in Moray compared to that of their peers living in cities.

People in Spey Bay are looking to build good lives in a place that is not only quiet and beautiful but also relatively cheap to live in compared to much of the rest of the country.[53] Some of them are just starting out, at the beginning of their careers, whilst some are starting again, after a relationship breakup, health problems, or unemployment.[54]

Spey Bay was also a haven for people's friends, who sometimes came to get away from their troubles in a place where they could treat each day as it comes. A friend of a friend of Sophie's came to stay with her after suffering a relationship breakup and a broken neck in a car accident and ended up staying three months. During a conversation with Sophie about this friend, she told me, "It's nice that coming to Spey Bay has made her start to think about settling down" and reflected that when she had come to Spey Bay herself in her mid-twenties, she realised that "although travelling is really good and fun, staying in one place, when it's the right place and you have a job you love and people you love, can be the really amazing thing." A good life is one that is both virtuous and enjoyable—the positive experience of intimate sociality is just as important as the area's beauty, pace of life, and closeness to the natural world.[55]

Friendship in Spey Bay is reminiscent of that between gay people in San Francisco as described by Kath Weston in her classic study. For some gays and lesbians, Weston argues, a relationship between friends or lovers that is envisaged to endure is expressed in terms of a "forever" that "represents neither a will to eternity nor an immutable biogenetic connection, but rather the outcome of the day-to-day interactions that organize a relationship." As she says, "In this transformation of the dominant biogenetic paradigm for kinship, permanence in a relationship is no longer ascribed ('blood is blood'), but produced."[56] As with the friendships between people here, it is the work that goes into making and maintaining them that becomes significant and that, in turn, makes the relationships ever more lasting and important.[57] People in Spey Bay did differentiate between kinship and friendship, suggesting that each relationship is characterised by different types of knowledge and that biogenetic kinship is supposed to bring a permanence that friendship may lack. Nonetheless, the intimate "warts and all" relationships that they have with their friends suggest both that this difference can be eroded to the point of meaninglessness and that kinship needs to be nurtured. So, whilst kin are supposed to always be there, all relationships are constantly made and remade. In Spey Bay, people's friends are the ones who give them support on an everyday basis and in times of trouble and who know their flaws as much as their strengths. They are also the ones people enjoy spending most of their time with. Friends are the people who will help out when the septic tank develops a blockage and they are the ones who will share a well-earned drink with you after you have cleared it.

Many people in Spey Bay cannot claim belonging to the place through birth, but their ties with other people and the land are still vital to the feeling of being at home there. This suggests the importance of choosing responsibly in their visions of a good life and the significance of care and effort in the present and future, rather than the privileges of birth and history. In order to have a life that is better, people in Spey Bay prioritise the place and what it has to offer over their native ties, but the relationships they have in that place are vital to the enjoyment of a good life. Many would be happy for the geographical distance between themselves and their families to be shorter, yet at the same time, a certain amount of distance allows them to select and reject elements of mainstream society in order to build lives in which a certain amount of difference is positively appreciated. Of course, even in those places where people do have primordial links at their disposal, their employment of them is by no means predictable or straightforward[58] and the facility to claim belonging or kinship using elements of both "given" and "made" knowledge is inherent in British models of kinship and identity.[59] For people in Spey Bay, it is the work and care that go into cultivating and conserving links between people, and between people and place, that are vital to maintaining good relationships, fostering a sense of belonging, and ultimately making a good life.

People in Spey Bay all take an interest in local issues, and those who have moved to Moray have made efforts to find out more about local history and culture, including attending folk music concerts and ceilidhs, trying Scottish food, and travelling around different parts of Scotland. But although they obviously think Scotland is a good place to make a good life, they tended not to fetishise Scottishness in the way that, for example, the North Americans, Australians, and South Africans with Scottish ancestors in Paul Basu's study of roots tourists to Scotland did.[60] There is, to be sure, anti-Englishness in Scotland, just as there is, like anywhere else, racism, sectarianism, homophobia, and sexism, but it is a minority pursuit. During my fieldwork in Spey Bay no one I knew was subject to any anti-English sentiment there, and in all the time I have spent working, travelling, and living in Scotland throughout my life, I have never experienced this kind of prejudice myself, though I know some who have. Although nationality is by no means a major focus of this book, it is, like anywhere else, part of the picture of life in Spey Bay. What should become clear is that there is fluidity to people's identities here, and this is probably facilitated in part by the fact that Scotland is both a nation with a well-established, and frequently romanticised, identity and part of the United Kingdom (and, beyond that, the European Union [EU]).

Having said this, it is increasingly difficult to take unity between the British nations (and for that matter between the UK and EU) for granted. On 18 September 2014, whilst writing this book, I stayed up until 5 a.m. the next day watching the results of what had been hailed as a historic decision for the future of the country: the Scottish referendum on independence from the UK. At the time of writing, it remains to be seen what effects—social, political, economic, and constitutional—the 55 percent majority decision to stay part of the UK, the enthusiasm for change that Scottish people expressed during the campaign, the promises to deliver more devolved powers to Scotland (and the other nations of the UK) by Westminster politicians, and the results of the UK General Election in May 2015 will each have on the Union's future. In the referendum, 57.6 percent of the residents of Moray voted to stay in the UK. Northeastern Scotland has traditionally been the stronghold of the Scottish National Party (SNP), which was the main political party pushing for independence, so in some ways it is surprising that there was not more enthusiasm for independence amongst the residents of Moray, though other traditionally SNP areas including neighbouring Aberdeenshire also voted "no," suggesting that the yes/no divide on independence did not in any simple way mirror party political allegiances.

The referendum on independence would never have been possible were it not for the SNP's increasing success at national elections, which came to a head during my fieldwork when, on 3 May 2007, after the third election since the establishment of the devolved Scottish Parliament, they emerged as the first party, just ahead of Labour, and formed a minority government with then leader Alex Salmond as the first minister. They went on to win a landslide victory in 2011, giving them the first majority government in the history of the contemporary Scottish Parliament and enough confidence to secure the referendum on Scottish independence in September 2014. Although I do not think that many people I knew in Moray voted for the SNP in the 2007 election, they did feel let down by the Labour government and then prime minister Tony Blair in the wake of the Iraq War and so felt some sympathy for the SNP as an alternative to Labour, given their left-of-centre and social-democratic political stance. Some also specifically expressed approval of Moray's SNP MP Angus Robertson's take on environmental issues.

Themes of nationality, belonging, connection, and identity recur in the poetry of John Mackie, whom I got to know during my fieldwork. John is in his sixties. He was born in Garmouth, the village on the opposite bank of the Spey to Spey Bay, where his mother lived until her death at age 101. John spent some of his childhood and much of his adult life in London, as well as living and working for some years in northern Africa. He returned to Moray with his wife, who was terminally ill, so that she could enjoy a healthier lifestyle in the final period of her life. After she died he decided to stay and he lives in Banff, Aberdeenshire, about a forty-minute drive from Spey Bay. In his poem "Ancestral Voices—A Polemical Rant on Scottish Identity," he draws on the scattered locations of his ancestors, which traverse Scotland, England, and North America like a genealogical spider's web. In the following passage, he expresses, through his ancestors, his own ideas about identity:

> As we sit late in our high house in Banff,
> once owned by a Polish grocer, ancestral voices
> silent in their frames speak volumes
> they say—Nationality is a construct, its foundations symbols
> of a shared, often mythical, past—Identity
> is more particular and proven.

John told me with some amusement that he had once recited "Ancestral Voices" at an informal SNP event and been told by audience members that it was a good example of nationalist poetry. Yet, in concluding, he reminds us that nationality, like any other aspect of identity, must be made and maintained through certain performances and rhetorical claims:

> we polish and practice
> the people we'll be:
> selecting from ancestral voices,
> fashioning diversity.

John's sense of the contingency of identity and belonging is particularly interesting given his status as a native of Moray with genealogical connections there that are clearly significant to him and that he could choose to foreground rather than question. What seems to be most important to him is the ongoing, and selective, feeling of connection in making identity and a sense of belonging. In her description of feeling at home in Spey Bay that I recounted earlier, Sophie identified three aspects of her daily experience: the place, the work, and the people. The primary affect that she associated with this was love. People in Spey Bay have an affective kinship with their friends, though they also feel and care for the environment in which they live; these feelings and the ways they are made on an everyday basis will be dominant themes throughout the coming chapters.

Caring for the Environment

Everyone knows Allan, a retired resident of Spey Bay, who is often out walking his dog and his neighbours' dogs too. Chris, my boyfriend at the time, had one notorious encounter whilst walking along the Spey in which Allan told him how fortunate he felt because his house, which overlooks the golf course, is "the highest house in Spey Bay" and so, he surmised, he would be the last remaining resident "when the seas rise." Allan observed that most other houses in the village are situated around sea level, whilst his is a whole four metres above the sea. When Chris got back from his walk and recounted this to our friends in Spey Bay they were largely amused, though one asked rhetorically, "And who is he expecting to row out to his little island with food and everything to keep him going when this happens?"

Allan's unsolicited comment about rising sea levels shows that climate change is a common concern amongst local residents, though people have different ideas about how they will be affected. The people who worked in the wildlife centre valued Allan as part of the local landscape, as "a character," but also as a compassionate man who cares about animals and tries to help other people, however eccentric some of his ideas might be. In their response to his comments about being the only survivor in Spey Bay after the seas rise, they bowed to his proprietorial and authoritative vision of the future but managed to retain a place for themselves in the image of them taking supplies to him in

rowing boats, a rather poignant one for people involved in cetacean conservation. Whilst they are prepared to respect, and even
prioritise, older and longer-standing residents' claims to belonging, this shows the importance they place on their attachment to
the place, such that they would not abandon it even in flooding,
and their self-appointed role caring for others.

When I have discussed and written about my time in Spey
Bay, people have often expressed surprise at the lack of conflict
in my accounts. It is something that surprises me, too, as I am
well aware of the fact that environmental campaigns can irri-
tate and alienate some people and that activism about the natural world can lead to conflicts between "local" and "incomer"
groups or "do-gooders." During fieldwork, I spent most of my
time with people who work in the wildlife centre and visitors,
who not surprisingly have sympathy for the cause of cetacean
conservation. So, through this association, I might simply have
missed out on being exposed to the other side of the argument.

One possible reason for the lack of noticeable conflict between conservationists and locals here is that Moray is a place
that attracts quite a few different incomers, who seem to settle
into the community successfully. It may also be something to do
with the specific case of Spey Bay: the wildlife centre is housed
in a building that already existed and that might otherwise become derelict, it is free for all to visit, it provides the only café in
the village, and visitors have little negative impact on the village,
tending to arrive in small numbers, drive slowly through the
village, and park their cars neatly in the wildlife centre car park.
The fact that the wildlife centre also encourages local people to
volunteer and that there are various initiatives to include local
residents in their work also probably goes some way to building
bridges. I did overhear local people referring to people from the
wildlife centre collectively as "the dolphin people" a couple of
times, which could be interpreted a number of ways, though I
think it was not intended to be derogatory. I am sure that there
are moments when people resent the fact that the wildlife centre
employs so many people who are not from the local area or feel

that they are being preached to. Nonetheless, where I attend to issues of conflict in this book, I focus much more on conflict within individuals than between them—that is, on the questions, dilemmas, and internal conflicts that characterise trying to make a good life, as this is what people talked about with me much more.

Based on the conversations I did have with people other than those who work and volunteer in the wildlife centre, anthropogenic climate change is a common concern in this part of the world, and this is perhaps another reason why there was a lack of obvious conflict between people in the community. Environmentalist values have become mainstream in the twenty-first century, and this has only intensified in the years since I began my fieldwork. Environmentalism waxes and wanes in political discourse and it has been somewhat eclipsed in recent years by the economic crisis, but the environment remains an important topic of discussion, not least since climate change has come to be accepted as scientific orthodoxy.

In Britain, environmentalism has undergone a shift in identity from the Green movement towards ethical living.[61] Ethical living is a social movement that arose towards the end of the last century, inspired by the Green movement and campaigns for "sustainable" living. It is a largely individualised movement in which people seek out information themselves about how to lead a more "ethical," or ecologically responsible, lifestyle. Ethical living is guided by the principle of using natural resources in a more environmentally sound or sustainable manner and treating producers better—this is a movement that calls for better business ethics and forms of consumption that do the least harm to people, animals, and the environment.[62] Adherents can decide for themselves how far they wish, and whether they can afford, to incorporate these principles into their everyday decisions, but major areas of consideration for those wishing to follow an ethical living lifestyle are the sourcing and provenance of food, reducing the use of fossil fuels through making fewer private car journeys, reducing and recycling household waste, using alternative forms of energy, reducing water usage, growing their own food, eating less (or no) meat, consuming Fairtrade brands, wearing ethical fashion, and using sustainable resources to build and equip homes.[63] People in Spey Bay did not refer to themselves as explicitly following the ethical living movement, but much of their everyday practice was based in exactly these considerations.[64] They also go beyond this by contributing to the cause of cetacean conservation, which could range from participating in litter picks on the beach to teaching children about the dangers of industrial pollution to carrying out wildlife surveys.

The obvious critique of ethical living is that it places too much emphasis on individual actions and lifestyle factors rather than on changing the structural conditions that create an ecologically unsustainable world. The longer-term goal of ethical living is one of harnessing consumer demand to effect change, as well as to inculcate "better" habits in increasing numbers of individuals and families (though some companies have been accused of "greenwashing" products by overstating their environmental credentials and ethical value). Ethical living could therefore be seen as a pragmatic attempt to change capitalism by talking back to it in its own language. We live in a consumer society so it is not surprising that we think about ethics in terms of consumption, just as in earlier times we thought about ethics more in terms of god, social respectability, or familial obligations. Ethical living is not radical, nor is it enough on its own, but it can be a part of a response to the challenges of a changing climate and exploitative business practices, not least in the way in which it raises awareness of issues like fossil fuel extraction, industrial farming, and sweatshop labour and in that it fosters an ethic that is more careful of others. Whilst ethical living can be, and repeatedly has been, criticised for pandering to middle-class preoccupations and being inaccessible to people with less flexibility in their spending power, the fact is that living a more "ethical" or environmentally friendly life can be financially, politically, and socially costly for anyone, precisely because the world is currently organised in an unsustainable and environmentally destructive manner.

Maria Puig de la Bellacasa describes this as an "age of ethics," in which both public debate and academic research have turned to focus on ethics.[65] As she says, this can mean that political problems become subsumed into the private domain and appear a matter of personal choice. Puig de la Bellacasa argues that we should "interrupt" the association between personal ethical engagement and the private sphere and do more to foster collective ethico-political commitments.[66] The environmentalist movement has, from its inception, been one driven by care, as encapsulated in the common phrase "caring for the environment." I will return to questions of care, particularly in relation to work and gender, in later chapters, but here I would like to draw attention, following Puig de la Bellacasa, to the point that caring can also be a form of critique.[67] So, whilst the ethicisation of life in this contemporary moment might, in some cases, be a move towards depoliticisation, this is not to say that there is no critical thinking behind such movements.[68] Caring for the environment can be about pointing out historical contingency, challenging the status quo, and creating alternative visions of the future, and therefore deeply political. Similarly, ethical labour like the work that is done in the wildlife centre in Spey Bay is implicitly critical in that it seeks to fill in gaps in both social awareness and political will.

The fact that environmentalism asks something of everyone, from individuals to governments to corporations, and that it posits a cause constitutive of, yet bigger than, humanity is one of the reasons it is so challenging. Environmentalism by its very nature is a globalised phenomenon that transgresses and transcends the subdivisions people make of their worlds. As Marilyn Strathern has pithily put it, "A crisis perceived as ecological contains all."[69] It is a challenge for scholars of environmentalism because it is difficult to know how to pin down something that crosses national, species, ecological, and disciplinary boundaries.[70] But then ethnographers have always studied economics and politics alongside kinship, cosmology, and ritual and so perhaps we are in fact fortuitously placed to study environmentalism, albeit in its local manifestations.[71]

Kay Milton, one of the early organising forces in the anthropology of environmentalism, describes environmentalism as a "social commitment" involved in a quest for a "viable future."[72] In the epigraph to her introduction to *Environmentalism: The View from Anthropology*, Milton quotes Timothy O'Riordan, who says, "Environmentalism is as much a state of being as a mode of conduct or a set of policies."[73] In this ethnography, I take the idea that environmentalism is a state of being, a mode of conduct (as well as a code for conduct), and a set of policies seriously, in relating how this group of people living in northeast Scotland make good lives. However, to describe them as environmentalists is, like any other label, somewhat misrepresentative. Some are so committed to the cause of animal welfare that they will make themselves vomit if they believe they have unwittingly eaten some animal-derived product. Some think that buying organic cow's milk for their child is their main priority in being an ethical consumer. Some believe that pandas are not worth saving because they are too far gone down the road to extinction. Some use contraception because they believe it is irresponsible to add to the world's population without proper planning. Calling someone an environmentalist does not necessarily tell us much about their gender politics or their take on foreign policy, let alone where they shop or how they vote. This is why I do not tend to locate the people I write about in this book in the environmental movement so much as in their geographical location. Spey Bay, as somewhere that represents both a good life and a place in which ethical labour is being done, is their ethical locus. What I am interested in exploring here is not so much what it means to be an environmentalist but what it means to be concerned about the future of nature, when nature is conceived as that which all species depend upon to survive and reproduce.

People in Spey Bay are a particularly interesting group to think and talk about reproduction with not only because they have an explicit interest in nature but also because they think about ethics on an everyday basis. They understand ethics to be less about abstract moral principles and more about quotidian decisions. Taking an approach of caring for the environment is not only about reducing harms to other species or preventing the pollution of the natural world but also about seeing the world—and their own place in it—in a particular way. Environmentalism posits a world in which people are connected to others because they live in interdependent and meaningful relationships with them. Caring for the environment is not about subduing or mastering nature but living with it in a way that will secure a good future for all.

A Merographic Map of the Book

Just as Spey Bay is a place where the river meets the sea, *Making a Good Life* is an exercise in bringing things into relation, or making connections. In this book, I employ Marilyn Strathern's[74] concept of merographic connections—a Western knowledge practice in which one domain of knowledge is brought into relation with another in order to better understand it—as a methodological and conceptual tool in order to trace the flow of ethical values, relations, and substances in people's thinking about reproduction. Indeed, Sarah Franklin argues, "Merographic thinking . . . is part of the conceptual equipment necessary to make IVF both thinkable and doable, indeed to make it workable at all."[75] Charis Thompson has described the "ontological choreography" that goes on in ART clinics, in which scientific and technological techniques dynamically combine with familial and conjugal relationships, gender politics, legal regulations, economic considerations, and clinical protocols. She says, "What might appear to be an undifferentiated hybrid mess is actually a deftly balanced coming together of things that are generally considered parts of different ontological orders (part of nature, part of the self, part of society)."[76]

In this chapter, I have introduced some of the main themes of the book—making a good life, nature, ethics, and reproduction—and started to sketch what life in Spey Bay is like. One further theme that runs through the book is context, which is something I wish to play with as much as to theorise. This chapter has started to map the context of Spey Bay by describing the place and the feeling of being there and outlining some of the issues that preoccupy its inhabitants. In discussing merographic connections, Strathern talks about contexts rather than environments (though environmentalism is one of the many examples she takes up in her exploration of the condition of being "after nature"). Both "environment" and "context" refer to the setting within which an entity operates or exists, but context has the added element of aiding understanding. As the *Oxford English Dictionary* puts it, context is "the circumstances that form the setting for an event, statement, or idea, *and in terms of which it can be fully understood*."[77] So it is that ethnographers see one of their main roles as making particular ideas and actions intelligible by putting them into context. One question that runs through the whole book is what it means to put things in context. In *After Nature*, Strathern explains that "the very desire to put facts 'into their context' is a merographic move. The context, by virtue of not being equivalent with the thing put into it, will 'illuminate' the thing from a particular angle (display one of its parts)."[78] The fact that things can always be put into context and that there are a multitude of available contexts, of varying scales and depths, creates a sense of plurality; it seems that each new context will generate a new sense of perspective.[79]

Each of the chapters in this book focuses on a particular aspect of reproduction. In chapter 1, this is the plans and aspirations for having children of the people who work in Spey Bay and do not have children. The chapter introduces the major theme of the "stable environment," a term that was used by one mother, Erin, to describe the best conditions in which to have a child but that also provides a crucible for thinking about the connections between reproduction and the environment and about gender and ethics. This chapter focuses particularly on the relationship between plans for parenthood and work and especially the effects of gender on both professional and parenting roles.

In this first ethnographic chapter, I introduce the term "ethical labour." Ethical labour refers to activities and actions that are guided by particular ethical principles. I describe it as the work of caring and it includes formal actions like working for charitable causes as well as everyday acts of ethical self-fashioning such as consuming "ethical" products and conscious ethical actions like disposing of waste responsibly, instructing others in ethical virtues, or choosing one particular action over another because it appears more ethical. The use of the word "labour" is a deliberate reference to the fact that all of these actions are carried out in a context of advanced capitalism and neoliberalism—many of these actions resist or subvert these political and economic values, yet they are also difficult to extricate from them. "Labour" also relates to the fact that ethics are constantly being made. Of course, in making ethical decisions, we draw upon ethical principles and values, but these values are no more static than the people who are guided by them. A good life is only finished (if at all) at death.

Chapter 2 carries the theme of the stable environment out into the wider world by considering what it means to care about stabilising the natural environment in the interest of future generations. Much environmentalist thinking and rhetoric are concerned with preventing environmental degradation in order to secure a better future. This indicates the importance of reproduction—in humans and other parts of the natural world—in caring for the environment and working to prevent climate change. In this chapter, I will look in depth at the concerns that people in Spey Bay had about humans putting ourselves at risk of endangerment by destroying our natural environments and becoming overreliant on technology to create children.

This chapter also shows the salience of nature and naturalness to how people in Spey Bay think about reproduction, ethics, the future, and the environment. This point is taken further in the subsequent two chapters, the first of which focuses on birth and becoming a parent and the second on the ethical dilemmas provoked by surrogacy. In chapter 3, I analyse the importance of ideas of nature to how people in Spey Bay think about gender differences in parenting and the ethics of care and responsibility in parenthood. As I discuss in chapters 3 and 4, one theme that emerged from my interviews with people in Spey Bay was a strong belief in the maternal bond, and in chapter 4 I discuss how this is challenged and complicated by surrogacy. Public debates in the UK have been characterised by a resilient sense that surrogacy presents unique ethical problems, and I show how for people in Spey Bay, ideas of naturalness act as ethical guides in navigating these problems. My aim in this chapter is also to articulate the nuance and willingness to sympathise with others that characterised people's responses to ART.

A thread that runs from chapter 4 into chapter 5 is community. Community is, for people in Spey Bay, part of a good life and it is something that is constantly made. People in Spey Bay find community in their shared ethical interests and values, and this has an effect on how they think of themselves as well as how they relate to the environment in which they live. Ethics is not only about doing the right thing as an individual but also about how they live their lives and what they want their lives to be. Ethnographies of Britain have demonstrated the importance of ideas of community in this country, nowhere more pertinently to this case than in Jeanette Edwards's book *Born and Bred*, which is rare in the attention it pays to what reproduction means to people's sense of how they relate, and are related, to others and in its emphasis on the ways in which attitudes to ART flow beyond individual or conjugal identities into local, regional, and national communities. In chapter 4 I discuss how ideas about altruism in surrogacy relate not only to individual ethical decision making but also to a sense of community and shared identity. In chapter 5, I extend the discussion of surrogacy by focusing on how people in Spey Bay thought about paying for bodily services and substances and what they felt this said about them as members of a community.

The final chapter is in some ways a conclusion, as it returns to the overarching themes of the book, yet it is not intended to sum up, so much as to suggest further shakes of the kaleidoscope. This is in keeping with the book's aim of showing, both in its content and its structure, that both life and ethics are constantly made but also a recognition of the fact that this book is just one, partial account of life in Spey Bay. This point is also reflected in the subchapters that come in between each chapter. These reflection sections, as I have come to think of them, are partly inspired by a similar narrative device used by Timothy Choy in his ethnography of Hong Kong environmentalism, *Ecologies of Comparison*. Whilst air was Choy's primary element, mine is water and so, like the constantly changing play of sunlight on water, these sections present other aspects of life in Spey Bay drawn from my observations, in turn suggesting new perspectives on the themes of the main chapters. These reflection sections also provide me with a space in which to consider the ethic, and ethics, of ethnography by reflecting on my own relations to Spey Bay and its various inhabitants. As Thom van Dooren[80] has observed, placing ourselves in the worlds we describe means we have a stake in them and may be held accountable for our accounts of them.

Making a Good Life examines what nature, ethics, and reproduction mean to people in Spey Bay whilst keeping these three aspects of life in constant contact. Each shifts in and out of focus like the pieces of a kaleidoscope, and some of the connections may seem absurd,[81] but the serious point I wish to get across is the preposterousness of treating reproduction as if it were separate from the rest of life. Merographic connections both describe and make contexts. They create a sense of plurality and diversity, but as Franklin has pointed out, there is also an "analogic return" in this process.[82] The meanings that are made through merographic connections travel back from one domain to the other with which they have connected, like waves cresting and hitting the shore. And just as when the river meets the sea, the potency of such connections lies not just in the internal logics of each domain but in the effects of their connection:[83] freshwater meets saltwater, salmon meets dolphin . . .

// Where the River Meets the Sea

John Mackie is a local who has returned to his "homeland"—as he puts it in his poem "Where the River Meets the Sea," he has "circled" back to Moray "like the Arctic Terns of the Spey." Through the example of his father's relationship to the Spey, in this poem, he considers the persistent dilemma of how best to live with the natural world:

> How long was his love for that river
> In its unbound abandon
> And the headlong salmon
> Soaring high from its spate
> And how broad his contempt
> For the efforts of those
> Who tried to impose
> The violence of order
> On its deep dark flow

I have always been struck by John's simple yet evocative description of Spey Bay as a place where the river meets the sea. Not only is the Spey a significant geographical feature and physical force, in that it literally shapes and shifts the ground on which Spey Bay is built, it is also the economic lifeblood of the place. The same could be said of the sea, and most people, when standing in Spey Bay at the mouth of the river, find their attention pulled by the swell of the tide, the drama, scale, and occasional sightings of marine mammals offered by the Moray Firth. Life in Spey Bay is characterised by the constant presence of water nearby. Both the river and the sea teem with life, though not as much life as before industrialised fishing or whaling. They support the lives of humans who live both nearby and further afield and they inspire relaxation, awe, and fulfilment. They are, also, places of danger and death, constant reminders of nature's force and of what is at stake in human activities that pollute the natural world and contribute to climate change. When people see dolphins in the firth or otters in the river, they provoke a surging feeling of hope and the poignant recognition of endangerment. This environment, and the good life it is thought to offer, is all the more precious because it might well be lost.

Having grown up near Cambridge, fifty miles from any coastline, then moving to London at age eighteen, during fieldwork I had to get used to the way that being so close to the sea changed not only my outlook but also my comportment. Small things, like tying my long hair back when I was outside so the wind wouldn't whip it into my face, reminded me constantly of the way in which the environment could affect me. Habitually faced with a roaring sea and biting wind, I had little sense that I had the power to master nature by virtue of my species.

Imagine, for a moment, Spey Bay viewed not from the land but from the water. After all, Spey Bay is not only the name of the village at the mouth of the Spey but also the bay itself, which ranges from Buckie in the east to Lossiemouth in the west. It is worth pausing for a moment and considering how the Moray Firth dolphins might perceive the efforts that some humans go to on their behalf—although perhaps they would be less interested in these activities than in how people think about and characterise them. Would they recognise the kinship between humans and themselves that people do? Would they value the intelligence and sociality that humans attribute to them as a species? And the Spey salmon—what do they sense when they get the impression of a human presence? Do they distinguish between an osprey flying overhead and the fighter jets of RAF Lossiemouth rending the sky as they practice their aerial manoeuvres?

Probably none of the questions would be meaningful to either the dolphins or the fish and I ask them precisely for that reason, in order to show how entrenched the separations that we imagine between people and the species with which we co-exist are and how fundamental certain ways of thinking and

particular values—intelligence, consciousness, altruism, kinship, identity—are to our perception of our environments and
ourselves. And yet I do not want to overstate this separation,
because otherwise I would not be able to pose these questions at
all. What they demonstrate is that there is space for us to cross
habitual boundaries, and thereby make a thinking dolphin
thinkable.

In his essay "Hunting and Gathering as Ways of Perceiving
the Environment," Tim Ingold discusses the persistent suppo-
sition that nature is a cultural construction.[1] As he makes clear,
whilst this in some ways moves the debate forward politically
and ethically, in that it allows for a somewhat less paternalistic
view of non-Western peoples, it carries within it Western assumptions about nature, reality, and the relationship of nature
to culture, specifically that there is a fundamental separation between nature and culture and that any attribution of consciousness or intention or other such "human" qualities to non-human
entities can only be metaphorical. Perhaps most important in
this, in that it limits us from seeing beyond these precepts, is
the assumption that, whatever is done with or upon nature, it is
still also an eternal and timeless presence. This idea of nature as
a given, pre-cultural grounding[2] is one that underlies the common elision of the environment with nature, particularly in the
phrase "the natural world," which I use in this ethnography as
an emic category, whilst also bearing in mind its uncanny ability
to seep back into analysis.

Ingold draws on the example of the comparison between
geese and people in Cree thought. He says,

> The point is that the difference between (say) a goose and a
> man is not between an organism and a person, but between
> one kind of organism-person and another. From the Cree
> perspective, personhood is not the manifest form of hu-
> manity; rather the human is one of many outward forms of
> personhood. And so when Cree hunters claim that a goose
> is in some sense like a man, far from drawing a figurative

parallel across two fundamentally separate domains, they are rather pointing to the real unity that underwrites their differentiation.[3]

Of course, people in Spey Bay do not hunt or gather their food, and catching salmon in the Spey is now the leisure activity of mostly middle-aged men who are legally obliged to comply with the terms of the fishing licences they have purchased. Nonetheless, as John's poetry articulates, this is a place where people are constantly compelled to consider their place in nature. Being part of the natural world rather than something that acts upon it is fundamental to the ethic of Spey Bay.

By attributing a speculative consciousness to the wildlife of Spey Bay, by applying a fish-eye lens, so to speak, I am not trying to imply that people there think about animals, landscape, or water in animistic ways. If anything, my aim is instead to evoke the discomfort of such boundary crossings, thereby demonstrating the tenacity of these separations, of human and animal, earth and water, culture and nature. It is also to suggest that the relations people have here with the natural world are not quite as separate or as differentiated as the mainstream models of nature within their own cultural milieu might suggest. In fact, just as people do not mechanically follow the highest moral ideals in making ethical decisions and judgements, there is also some slippage between what counts as human and what counts as non-human. So, although the people who work in the wildlife centre roll their eyes at depictions of smiling dolphins frolicking under rainbows, they do, in many ways, see eye to eye with cetaceans. Like everything, it depends on the context.

The first time I met John, I had just watched him recite some of his poetry in a public performance in Spey Bay icehouse. He finished with one of his older poems, "Whalesong." He was accompanied on acoustic guitar and made full use of the microphone and the submarine-like acoustics of the icehouse to make his voice as resonant as possible. Over the following months, John became increasingly involved in the work of the wildlife

centre. On a return trip to Spey Bay in 2008, I had a conversation with him about his poetry as we sat by the beach looking
out to sea. He had recently been on a local wildlife-watching
cruise. "I think of 'Whalesong' now as my 1970s poem, because
it draws on this cultural notion that whales are sacred," he told
me, before adding, "I wonder sometimes if whales and dolphins
have taken the place of medieval gods." I smiled at this, appreciating John's habitual mixture of erudition and playfulness.
This provocative speculation was no doubt also an attempt to
get me to divulge my own opinion about the cultural meanings
of cetaceans. I didn't rise to his bait, so he continued, "I'm going
to rewrite it, now I've been on this trip. The skipper gradually
disabused us of all this New Age stuff. For example, you think
you've seen a lovely leap in the air, but it's four males gang-
banging a female. That's what we need to remember instead of
all this sacred stuff—it's biological. I want to rewrite it with the
marine biology facts in it."

Human conceptions of the earth and how we are situated
in, with, or upon it are closely related to our politics and ethics[4]
and to our relations with others, whatever their species.[5] By suggesting that we pause to look back at Spey Bay from the sea, I
want to question the idea that we should draw the line of our
attention at the water's edge and to educe a sense of being part
of the natural world rather than something that acts upon it.
Doing fieldwork can feel like being underwater, with nothing
but slippery fronds of seaweed to hold onto. It can make you feel
vulnerable, lost, endangered, and all too aware of your limitations. But that sense of being unable to breathe also reminds us
of just how dependent on our environments we are.

Ethical Labour

Why, hopelessly and romantically, do we imagine
a natural preserve of feeling, a place to be kept
"forever wild"? The answer must be that it
is becoming scarce.

—*Arlie Russell Hochschild*

In This Day and Age

When I joined Joanna and Sophie for breakfast in the wildlife centre café one Sunday morning, I knew from their animated faces that something had happened. Sophie quickly told me that Joanna, a health care assistant and wildlife centre volunteer in her mid-twenties, had just found out that her teenaged sister, Gemma, was pregnant. It was clear that Joanna disapproved of her sister's actions. She seemed most concerned about their mother, whom she felt would be the one to pick up the pieces. Joanna explained as we ate our breakfast that what frustrated her most about Gemma's pregnancy was that it was planned. She told us this with characteristic openness and paid little attention to whether the other diners heard her, but suddenly lowered her voice to a whisper when she added, "She even went off the Pill."

Joanna's disapproval was primarily motivated by concern and care—for her sister, her parents, and her future niece. As she got used to the idea, however, she became excited and happy for her sister and was as supportive as she could be, given that they lived five hundred miles apart. Joanna, like her colleagues and friends, believed that people should plan to have children when they are ready. Her initial reaction to her sister's decision to become a mother whilst she was still legally a child herself reflected her judgement that Gemma lacked the maturity, sense of responsibility, and resources to be a *good* mother. Because of her youth, Gemma's choice to become a mother was not viewed as an index of her readiness but quite the opposite.

I came across another, stronger reaction of disapproval to an "inappropriate" pregnancy whilst chatting with Margaret, a Spey Bay resident in her sixties who originally comes from Perthshire, in the wildlife centre one afternoon. She spotted Paula, a single mother and waitress in her mid-twenties who lives in Spey Bay with her parents and preschool daughter, in the distance.

"Is Paula pregnant again?" Margaret asked me in a hushed voice. The word "pregnant" was barely audible. I nodded. "Does she have a steady boyfriend?"

"I don't know," I replied, though I was fairly sure she did not.

"In this day and age, *ken*?[1] Unbelievable," Margaret said, shaking her head.

Not long afterwards, the same subject came up in conversation with Willow, a member of the wildlife centre staff in her mid-twenties. She also asked me if I knew whether Paula was in a relationship but caught herself and added, "That's an awful question to ask, I know."

//

People in Spey Bay rarely brought up ideas of inheritance in the sense of either phenotype or property when I talked with them about reproduction, but they did share the sense that future generations will inherit the environments that they create. This is encapsulated, in a practical sense, by their assumption that parental responsibility begins with planning and creating a "stable environment" for children to be born into. This term, which was coined by Erin, who is married with a daughter, describes the ideal conditions in which to become a parent. Her deeply resonant phrase eloquently condenses her aspirations and anxieties for future generations, which were shared by everyone I knew in Spey Bay. The stable environment parents are expected to create for their children includes financial security, being in a happy relationship, emotional maturity, and a willingness to take on the responsibilities and sacrifices of parenthood. This reflects an ethic that children should be planned for and that ideally they will be conceived in a context that is conducive to their physical and emotional well-being and that will also enable their parents to be "good" parents. This resonates with middle-class ideals about good parenting and the assumption that reproductive decision making needs to be balanced against parents' careers.

The idea of the stable environment runs through this book, but it is particularly prominent in this chapter and the next one. In this chapter, I will explore people's ideas about good parenting by focusing on how those who do not have children plan for parenthood by creating a stable environment for their future children. In the next chapter, I will broaden the focus by looking at how conceptions of the environment and the state of the natural world are implicated in people's ideas about parenthood, fertility, and future generations. This chapter will also continue the scene-setting of the introduction, so I will describe the work that goes on in the wildlife centre before discussing the plans for future parenthood of those staff members who did not have children, both of which can be seen as forms of ethical labour. Later in this chapter, I will dwell on the concept of ethical labour to explore the links between profession and parenthood in more depth.

This chapter takes the connection between career aspirations and planning for parenthood seriously by tracing the relationship between the professional and parental ethics of the people with no children who live and work in Spey Bay. As I will discuss further in chapter 3, although people in Spey Bay were supportive of gender equality at work, they did assume that women would be the primary caregivers of children, so their careers would be most affected by parenthood. Charity work is a female-dominated form of labour, and this is reflected in the staff of the wildlife centre in Spey Bay, which is mostly made up of women. Charity work is also popularly seen as a feminine field, in which values of care, altruism, flexibility, and dedication go alongside a blurring of professional and personal boundaries and identities, so this is a fruitful form of work to consider alongside women's aspirations for future motherhood.

Doing a Good Job

Every hour during daylight in the summer months, a wildlife centre staff member stands, dressed in warm clothing branded with the conservation charity's logo, on the small mound by the icehouse with a pair of powerful binoculars and a stopwatch, clipboard, and pencil. After scanning the sea for ten minutes, she records the time, visibility, sea state (on the Beaufort scale), type, and number of birds and boats visible and any dolphin, seal, whale, or porpoise sightings, by number, the amount of time for which they were visible, and their behaviour. This is Shorewatch, the hands-on research that they do at Spey Bay and one of the jobs I did regularly as a volunteer.

Dolphins are much more commonly sighted in the summer, not only because that is when they tend to be feeding in the shallower bays of the inner Moray Firth but also because the seas are usually calmer so they are easier to spot. Typically the first sign for dolphin-watchers is a dorsal fin cutting through the water. Since bottlenose dolphins are grey (though they appear almost black from a distance) and the sea has a rather greyish hue, they can be quite difficult to spot, but once seen they are unmistakeable, especially if they then begin to hunt or "play," leaping through the air, throwing fish, or slapping the water with their tails. Usually dolphin sightings, being unpredictable, happened outside the allotted minutes of Shorewatch. At these times, a rush of excitement would pass through the wildlife centre as word spread that dolphins had been spotted.

In Spey Bay, it was difficult to avoid having conversations about dolphins and whales with locals and visitors alike. Indeed, whilst in the field, cetaceans seeped into my mind so deeply that I regularly dreamed about them. Quite a few villages along the Moray Firth coast have dolphins painted on local signs or in the decoration of shops, and locally made greetings cards often display photographs of dolphins taken in the firth. It is also common for people to hang small blue plastic dolphin figures from their car rearview mirrors. Dolphins and whales are often on the minds of people in Moray. In fact, when I first met one wildlife centre employee and described my interest in reproductive technologies, she replied quite matter-of-factly, "Oh, did you know, dolphins do surrogacy? When the babies are born the females take turns to look after them."

The conservation charity that runs the wildlife centre in Spey Bay employs six full-time paid staff based in the centre plus two who are not office based and two more in its smaller sister centre near Inverness that opened in 2007. During the summer, they employ around five residential volunteers (this was extended to cover the winter season as well after I left the field). Residential volunteers, who stay for about six months, are provided with accommodation and a weekly food allowance and many told me that part of the appeal of working at Spey Bay was that, unlike many overseas conservation projects, they did not have to contribute towards their living costs to work there. Most of these volunteers were recent graduates in their twenties, from the UK or Western Europe, but a few were also in their thirties or forties, taking "career breaks" or trying something new. Non-residential volunteers are called "local volunteers" and they typically give about a day a week of their time to helping out in the wildlife centre and at events. They include students getting work experience in conservation, retired or school-age locals from Spey Bay and neighbouring villages, and recent incomers to the area who support the cause and are interested in meeting new people. The charity, whose headquarters is based in southwest England but which has four more international offices, also part-funds a scientific research project with Aberdeen University on the Black Isle, on the other side of the Moray Firth, and volunteers and staff typically participate in annual surveys of the local cetacean population run by this team.

The public area of the wildlife centre is made up of the shop, café, icehouse, wildlife garden, and exhibition area, which also serves as a location for talks and a children's play area. There is also an office, storeroom, and volunteer accommodation on site. The exhibition area is reached through the shop and consists of a series of interpretation boards with information about the Moray Firth dolphins, local wildlife, climate change, and animal conservation. It is also the location of the sightings board, where staff members record the most recent wildlife sightings at Spey Bay and elsewhere nearby. The rest of the exhibition is in the separate icehouse, usually only open in the summer as it is prone to flooding in wet weather, where visitors are shown a DVD about whales and dolphins, given a talk on the history of Spey fishing, and shown historical fishing equipment. In the shop they sell books, soft toys, gifts, ornaments, and clothes branded with the charity's logo or with pictures of wildlife on them, as well as some locally flavoured items such as folk music CDs by local bands, tea towels printed with humorous ditties about Scotland, and guides to the local area.

During summer, the centre is open seven days a week, whilst in winter it is only open on weekends. On a typical summer day, some of the paid staff will be working in the office, whilst the education officer might be leading a school group. At least one residential volunteer will be guiding on a wildlife-watching boat out from neighbouring Buckie. Either a paid employee or residential volunteer will be in charge of the shop, supported by one or more local volunteers, who keep in touch with staff in the office via walkie-talkies. Other staff members, often volunteers, will also be running regular talks in the exhibition space such as a guide to the best places to spot dolphins, with an emphasis on promoting reputable tour operators, as well as hourly tours of the icehouse. One staff member will also be on rota doing Shorewatch.

Wildlife centre staff had daily direct contact with supporters and members of the public, which they saw as an opportunity to educate people about the threats faced by cetaceans, focusing particularly on the Moray Firth dolphins, and to promote the interests and causes of the charity as a whole. Many local school parties visit the centre during the spring and summer months to take part in educational activities hosted by them. I helped out on many of these occasions, assisting children in making sea-themed musical instruments, participating in games that illustrate the importance of recycling rubbish, and leading nature trails along the banks of the Spey. Staff members also travel to local sites for special events. Such events are multipurpose, providing opportunities for fund-raising, education, advocacy, and the promotion of environmentally responsible behaviour in the local population.

Thousands of visitors come to the wildlife centre each year, lured by the opportunity of seeing dolphins, ospreys, seals, and other wildlife in their natural habitats. The two main groups who visit the centre are families with young children and naturalists (which includes birdwatchers as well as cetacean-watchers), but it also appeals to passing tourists who do not have a specific interest in cetaceans. A large number of visitors are holidaymakers from England, and many of these are repeat visitors to Spey Bay and the wildlife centre. Many locals also visit the centre, either by themselves or with visiting friends and family, including especially children and grandchildren. The centre is well-known locally and has in a sense put the village on the map. A sizeable proportion of visitors I met whilst volunteering in the centre expressed great affection for the place and saw a visit there as a treat, for adults and children alike.

Behind the scenes, staff members are positive about visitors and many were adept at drawing people into friendly conversations and making them feel welcome by listening attentively to accounts of their experiences wildlife-watching or their holiday plans. Since the centre is small and often has quiet periods with only a few visitors present, there is time to talk to people and so

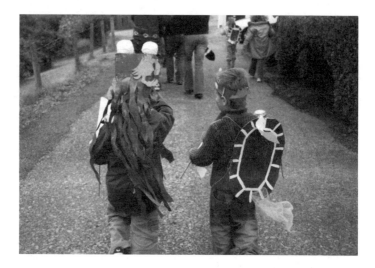

Figure 4. Children take part in an annual Save the Whale parade in Spey Bay, dressed in sea creature costumes made by them earlier in the day. Photo by author.

create a sense that they are being personally attended to. As the centre is free to visit, staff members were also very open about recommending other places to visit to tourists, since they did not see themselves in competition with other sites, as the wildlife centre is unique in the area.

One cause of consternation amongst centre staff, though, was the relative regularity with which visitors would come into the centre and ask where they keep the dolphins, as if it were a dolphinarium. There are no dolphinariums in the UK because, although they are not illegal as such, the animal welfare regulations are so restrictive as to make them unviable, and one of the main points that staff members in the centre are keen to get across to visitors is that capturing and keeping cetaceans for public exhibition is, in their view, cruel. Staff members see educating people about cetacean welfare as one of their main roles and they produce literature, which they give out for free in the wildlife centre, that argues that keeping them in captivity drastically reduces their life span and quality of life. The misperception of visitors and potential visitors that they might be running a dolphin captivity programme at Spey Bay is exasperating for them, as it is a fundamental misunderstanding of what they stand for and it demonstrates that there is still a lack of awareness about the problems of keeping cetaceans in captivity amongst the general public. Whilst telling me about such visitors who had asked about seeing dolphins in captivity at Spey Bay, one staff member said to me, "We don't keep dolphins in tanks like SeaWorld! You have to come and watch and wait, you can't just expect to get everything you want whenever you want it!"[2]

As an alternative to seeing dolphins and whales in captivity, the wildlife centre promotes "responsible" wildlife-watching from small boats that do not "harass" wildlife. The wildlife-watching industry is growing steadily in the area, benefitting not only from an apparently ready market but also from the infrastructure of the local fishing industry. The wildlife-watching trips on which the Spey Bay volunteers guide are on a repurposed lifeboat led by a former fisherman and his wife, and a number of other tour operators have adapted fishing boats for wildlife cruises and operate out of the many local harbours that would once have been filled with fishing boats.

The presence of wildlife is also an important selling point for local tourism more generally. The Moray Firth coast is dotted with bed and breakfasts, hotels, guesthouses, and quite a few caravan and camping sites with mobile homes perched on the edges of the coast so as to maximise the sea views, which (mostly British) tourists stay in over the summer. Quite a few families in Spey Bay make the most of the local landscape and wildlife in their own business enterprises including the family that runs the café in the wildlife centre. Not surprisingly, although the café is technically a separate venture from the conservation charity, it is decorated with many depictions of dolphins including stencils of leaping dolphins on the walls. They also display for sale some of the artwork of a local retired couple, originally from Yorkshire, whose house in Spey Bay is crammed with their various arts and crafts projects, all of which in some way reflect the local environment but especially the sea. Margaret, who asked me above about Paula's relationship status, and her husband run a bed and breakfast that is explicitly sold to visitors on the promise of seeing dolphins, as the upstairs sitting room has an enormous full-length window that overlooks the bay and so provides ample opportunities for warm, comfortable dolphin-watching.

Making a Stable Environment

The idea of the stable environment indicates the importance of location and a sense of home in people's ideas about reproduction and parenting. Rural areas of Scotland have higher birthrates compared to those of cities, and Moray has one of the highest rates in Scotland, along with neighbouring Aberdeenshire and the Shetland Isles.[3] According to the Scottish Government, some of this may be "driven by selective migration of people wishing to start or increase their families from cities to suburban areas as a result of housing market and quality of life issues."[4] The people I lived amongst in Spey Bay certainly see Moray as a good place in which to bring up children, and many of their ideas about what makes a good life are coterminous with those about what makes a stable environment in which to parent. Access to beautiful landscapes and fresh air, proximity to the seaside, and opportunities to spot rare wildlife were seen as beneficial to both children and adults. The fact that people could afford to live in whole houses, often with their own gardens, on public and charity sector salaries was also valued. People assumed that having children takes a certain amount of money, and whilst they did not believe that children needed to be "spoiled" with luxurious toys and gifts, they did think that financial stability is part of being a good parent.

Ideas about community were also important in people's aspirations for their (future) children. Erin, who grew up in

Ireland and England, observed that people in Moray have "community spirit," which she thought people from other parts of the country might equate with a lack of sophistication. She said she thought that people in this area were "far more trusting with their children." She often mentioned to me that she had observed mothers leaving their children in pushchairs outside the village shop whilst they went in to buy something. She said that this worried her and that she would never do it herself but that she had come to understand that "it doesn't come out of ignorance, it comes out of a belief that children are loved and respected as part of the whole community and no 'normal' person would harm a child, so they feel safe to do that." In assessing this risky parenting practice, Erin, who had been a psychiatric nurse before having her daughter, showed her understanding of the community's values. Even though she could not quite bring herself to participate in it, she thought that the wider value of love and respect for children was something to be celebrated and that it made this a good place to be a parent.

During my first summer in Spey Bay, I attended a birthday party for Charlotte, a member of staff in the wildlife centre, at a pizza restaurant in Elgin. Her colleague Heather lived in Fochabers with her partner and was just about to leave her job at the wildlife centre to start a PhD in marine science. Whilst talking about this change of direction in her career during dinner, Heather suddenly brought up the subject of when she should start thinking about having a baby. She expressed the difficulty of juggling her enthusiasm about her studies, and the future job opportunities they might lead to, with her desire to become a mother. Willow said quite firmly that she could not imagine herself having a baby without being married first. Willow is a practising Christian, so I asked if this desire to be married first was to do with her religion. She said, "No, I just can't really see one [a baby] without the other [a husband]." She then turned to Charlotte, who lived with her partner, Mark, and joked that she would probably be pregnant within the year.

Charlotte laughed and admitted that she had been "feeling broody" for about six months.

The ubiquity of public debates about how people have children in the UK reflects changes in demography and reproductive and sexual practices, as well as greater acceptance of "alternative" family forms. With increasing use of contraception and the development of ART, parenthood has come to be seen as being chosen, or even achieved.[5] The idea that one can make conscious choices about reproduction reflects expectations about individual autonomy, as well as ideas about the human capacity to control "nature" and "biology."[6] The assumption that parenthood is now chosen and planned rather than an inevitable occurrence suggests that parenthood is therefore properly a site of ethical deliberation. If women choose to become mothers, then they may feel an extra responsibility to ensure that they have considered the implications of that choice.[7] These young women's deliberations about future motherhood over pizza reflect the taut balance between choice and expectation for middle-class women of their generation. Whilst they believe that they possess the autonomy to choose whether and when to have children, they were aware that this must be weighed against specific expectations about nature, time, age, and the connections between them.

Willow arrived in Spey Bay as a residential volunteer but, like Sophie, had stayed on after securing a paid job. Originally from England, she had moved to Scotland with her parents and younger siblings as a teenager, where they had settled. Before she arrived in Spey Bay in her mid-twenties, she had completed a degree in zoology and worked on a few conservation projects abroad. She eloquently articulated the tension between choice and expectation for women of her generation, based on her own experience:

> Well, it's difficult because I think our generation is quite lucky in some ways, 'cause we have got all these opportunities. I know that my mum said that when she was at uni., she had a choice of either doing nursing or teaching, and now we've

got a lot more choice. So we've . . . suddenly been opened up to all these possibilities, but at the same time, we're hemmed in by biology [*laughs ironically*], so it's really hard. We go and get educated and we think, "Well, hey, we want to do something with that now," but at the same time, you know, you have to start having kids at some point. But I can totally understand why people are having kids later. By the time my parents were my age they were married. I think they would be a bit shocked if I turned round and said I was getting married, you know, they'd be, "Oh, you're far too young!"

Gay Becker found in her study of infertile American couples that they experienced a crisis as they came to terms with the sense that their lives diverged from cultural norms and collective images of the human life course, and specifically the "core cultural construct . . . that biological reproduction is an automatically occurring event, one that is part of the natural order of life."[8] Many of Willow's colleagues and friends also related their own plans for parenthood to the experience of family and friends, suggesting that having children is a stage in an expected life course and that individual lives follow roughly congruent, linear trajectories in line with other cultural ideas about progress,[9] though some expressed concern about people being under pressure to have children. Sophie said, "I do think it's important that life—an individual's life—is not valued purely on whether they can reproduce or not." Sophie also told me that she had recently become more positive about future motherhood. She felt she had been more "selfish" and more inclined to "rebel from the norm" when she was younger and that that had influenced her sense that she did not want to have children. But as she had reached her late twenties, she had started to feel that she could in fact "imagine such a tie . . . [and] a future with that kind of responsibility." She concluded, "I think I feel a bit more, now, that what is most important is being able to care for [children] and that's something I feel a bit more able to do."

People in Spey Bay expected that most women would want to pursue their own careers and that this would be their priority in their twenties and thirties, leading them to "delay" motherhood until later in life. They were aware that later pregnancy is linked with higher rates of infertility and greater incidences of certain conditions such as Down Syndrome in children, but they were sympathetic to people having children when they are older as they also thought that, in a sense, parenting should start before a pregnancy is established, with the parents getting ready for the responsibilities that parenthood would bring about. Of course, such choices are enabled by the older reproductive technology of contraception. One afternoon, I was drinking tea in Sophie's sitting room with Lauren, who had just finished work for the day. Lauren was living with her partner and they were both in their late twenties at the time. Lauren was adamant that she was not yet ready to have children. She explained, "If I can't have a dog, then I certainly can't have a baby! That's the way I feel about it—I'm not stable enough to have a puppy, no baby either." As we discussed her future plans for parenthood further, it became clear that however unstable she felt, she had put a great deal of thought into becoming a mother one day. Lauren explicitly linked her fertility with time, reflecting on how long it might take between deciding she was ready, getting pregnant, and giving birth. She said, "Basically best scenario would be a year . . . until you have your child, and for most people that's not the case, particularly with the amount of birth control that we've all had, sort of—'forced down our throats' is a little bit violent—but there's . . . all the reasons why you may not conceive as quickly as you might, and [especially] if you're starting at a later age."

Lauren suggested that part of the choice to "delay" parenthood, and particularly motherhood, amongst people of her generation reflected a desire to, as she put it, "pre-set" their lives, so they had everything in place before having children, "rather than having a kid is what you do with your life and [everything] builds around that." Lauren's colleague and friend Amy told me that she had recently started to feel more certain about her desire to be a mother in the future, which she explicitly linked with turning thirty and with seeing her friends starting to have children. Like Willow and Sophie, Amy had worked and travelled in a number of different places before arriving in Spey Bay as a volunteer and, later, a paid member of staff. Like them, she saw Spey Bay as the place in which she had first felt she could "settle down" and start to build a home. In talking about her plans for future parenthood, Amy also reflected on the differences between a friend who had had an unplanned pregnancy and herself. She said that whilst her friend did not regret having her child, she thought she might have regretted "giving up a bit of her freedom," whereas Amy had had the opportunity to travel and work in different jobs and so, she concluded, "When I do have children, I think I'll be ready for them."

As the concept of the stable environment indicates, people in Spey Bay expected parenthood, and particularly motherhood, to bring about a unique sense of responsibility and they assumed that good mothering entails certain sacrifices as well as a reorientation of the self away from "selfishness" to altruism. Given this, it is unsurprising that many of the women I spoke to who had not had children felt that they should make the most of their opportunities to travel, establish their careers, or simply try different things before "settling down" into parenthood. Sophie pointed out that this is also an act of ethical labour. She said, "I suppose the variety of reasons why people might decide to delay having kids are so vast and it may be something that's absolutely critical for them to feel like they could support a kid in the future, and in that case, they're really trying to do something good."

Nina studied at Edinburgh University and worked on a conservation project in the Pacific before getting involved in the work of the conservation charity in Spey Bay. At the time that I interviewed her, her older sister had recently given birth to her first child, which she described as making her feel "very broody." She was the only young woman to dissent from the assumption that delaying motherhood to build a stable environment was the best thing to do, based on what she thought was most natural:

> I mean naturally, our bodies are ready to have children when we're younger and I think women feel this [pressure to] have a career and succeed in the same way that men are and so having children is sort of put on the back burner, I guess. I think being a young mum is good, I think it can be good for a child to have a young mum. I don't think being an older mum is bad, that's not what I'm saying, but I don't think it's a bad thing to have your children early and I think a lot people think it is, if you haven't had a career first and had that sort of achievement in your life, that you're doing something wrong.

Because more women than men work in the wildlife centre and those men who do work there tend to be older and already have children, I was not able to talk to many young men about their plans for parenthood. However, the younger men I spoke to who did not have children tended to be somewhat more relaxed about future parenthood than did their female peers. Lauren had clearly put quite a lot of thought into future motherhood, despite the fact that at the time she was adamant that she was not yet ready to have a puppy, let alone children. Like Amy, she was at a stage in her life when her friends were starting to have children, and she said that this had provoked her to reflect on how long it might take between deciding she was ready, getting pregnant, and giving birth. When I asked Lauren's partner, Jack, who was unemployed at the time, about his plans for fatherhood he observed that many people now want to have everything set up before having children and said that he would like that himself. But he told me that his older sister had had an unplanned pregnancy in her late twenties and then established her career in her mid-thirties, so because he had seen that that could work he was less concerned about planning for fatherhood compared to Lauren, who was prompted to reckon her future motherhood out year by year.

Richard and Paul both already have adult children, and when I interviewed them they each described realising they needed to become responsible when their first children were born. This contrasts with the aspiration of most of the younger people (but particularly women) in Spey Bay without children, who would prefer to have everything in place *before* they have a child. They want to be adults before they become parents rather than as a result of having children. Many expressed a sense that this was a generational shift, and Lauren suggested that people are "probably allowed to be children longer, nowadays." Younger people expected to be able to make their own decisions about when they became parents, not only because of a sense of autonomy but also because they feel that one should be a responsible adult in order to become a responsible parent. Whilst house prices and the general cost of living are lower in northeast Scotland than much of the rest of Britain, younger people envisaged financial strains when they did come to settle down. They felt that they should therefore build their careers not only for personal fulfilment but also to provide for their future dependants. Creating a stable environment is seen to take time and money, and if this has not been taken into account, there is a risk of being labelled a bad parent. And yet whilst a stable career might be necessary for a middle-class woman wanting to be a "good" mother, this assumption will be overturned once she becomes a mother because of the expectation that she will have primary responsibility for child care, as I discuss in chapter 3.

The idea of the stable environment condenses both the costs and rewards of parenthood. It contains tensions and contradictions in its own fabric and reveals much about people's ideas about what parenthood means and entails. The stable environment symbolises a point at which the main caregiver, who in a heterosexual couple will usually be the mother, will reorient her focus, reassess her sense of self, and rethink her priorities. It suggests that, before becoming parents, both men and women will pursue projects of self-fulfilment and actualisation, which are then rerouted into their children. This points to the importance of thinking of others in the ethical values of people in Spey Bay and in parenthood and reproduction but also the tacit recognition that their efforts to build good lives are *both* self-interested and other-oriented. In contrast to popular discourse that links greater choice with individualism and consumerism, the act of planning to become a parent is here linked with a reorientation of the self towards responsibly prioritising others' needs, yet in fact this orientation is not a sudden departure from childishness or selfish individualism, since people in Spey Bay already practise ethical labour, driven by values of care, goodness, and community, on a daily basis.

Caring

Whilst caring relationships are typically viewed as havens in a heartless world, care is also intimately tied to relations of domination and exploitation. It is activated by relations of dependency and relies upon individuals recognising and acting upon a sense of responsibility. The fact that women have historically worked in invisible or undervalued positions of care within the domestic sphere and that the ability to care is thought to come naturally to them has only contributed to a devaluing and dismissal of care in social life.[10] Thinking about caring work and professional work that is premised on an ethic of care illuminates the complexities and challenges that care presents to gender norms and hegemonic ideas about the nature of work.

During the last century, Marxists and feminists attempted to improve the lot of women by having their unpaid domestic and caring labour recognised as a form of work akin to that done by men in factories, on farms, and in offices. In the capitalist model that they were critiquing, men were productive and women reproductive; women's labour in the home was fundamentally enabling of men's waged work outside of the home.[11] The underlying premise of this model posited two antipathetic yet codependent spheres: the public world of work, which was rational, organised, and profit driven, and the private world of home, love, and family. But since the 1970s, work has changed, with declining numbers of full-time, permanent positions available and increasing casualisation and "flexible" labour, in which employees are more reliant on themselves and more vulnerable to changes in circumstances. More middle-class women are participating in paid work, and they are doing so not only because they believe they are equally capable of doing a job as a similarly qualified man but often also because they cannot afford to stay at home. This leaves a gap in care, which many solve by employing others to take on the domestic work of the household, typically on informal contracts.

In her classic work on emotional labour, Arlie Hochschild describes how an ethic of care has been put to work in the late capitalist economy. Hochschild defines emotional labour as that which "requires one to induce or supress feeling in order to sustain the outward countenance that produces the proper state of mind in others."[12] The rise of the service economy has gone along with increasing female participation in the workforce and, as Hochschild notes, emotional labour has been an important "resource" for women who have typically found it easiest to secure employment in jobs that require this, because good emotion management is popularly thought of as both a skill and a predisposition of women. Along with increasing numbers of people, and especially women, being employed in the service economy, there has been a professionalisation and commodification of "good service," which is epitomised in Hochschild's work by the public personae of flight attendants who must constantly maintain a sense that they are committed to meeting air passengers' needs, not because it is their job but because it is what they truly love doing. Yet Hochschild sees the move towards commercialised emotional labour as leading to a romanticisation of true, authentic feeling: "We are intrigued by the unmanaged heart and what it can tell us. The more our activities as individual emotion managers are managed by organizations, the more we tend to celebrate the life of unmanaged feeling."[13]

Drawing on the literature on the ethic of care, Hochschild's concept of emotional labour, and Cooper and Waldby's recent analysis of clinical labour,[14] I describe the work in the wildlife centre in Spey Bay as a form of ethical labour. Care consists of three intertwined and interrelated elements: an affective state, the recognition of ethical obligations, and practical actions.[15] Ethical labour is the work of caring: caring for the environment, caring about and for other people, caring about the future as manifested in the results of your work. In the context of work, it is caring about doing a good job and caring for the job you do. Since the 1980s, when Hochschild was writing, the commercialisation of emotions and the blurring of the boundary between professional and private self have only increased. This blurring is demonstrated by the case of charity work, which despite being avowedly different from the private and commercial sectors in that it is not profit driven is by no means immune to mainstream ideologies of professionalism, marketing, and accountability. Furthermore, the realities of working for charity are very much in line with the post-Fordist model of flexible, informal, and precarious employment that has become integral to twenty-first-century capitalism.

The good lives that people in Spey Bay are making are both ethically sound and emotionally fulfilling, and this double meaning of goodness is also the aspiration for their work lives. Doing work that you love is a middle-class ideal in the UK. Embedded in this ideal is an assumption that work—or at least the work most people do—is by its nature something that you would not usually choose to spend your time doing, were you not being paid for it.[16] Those who do paid work that they love can then feel that they are "beating the system," which may, ironically, make them more willing to tolerate periods of unemployment, long hours, low pay, and precariousness.

For middle-class people in Britain, a person's career is thought to say something about the kind of "real," private individual he or she is. Working for charity blurs the boundaries between the professional and personal and the public and private since choosing to work for a specific charity implies personal commitment to the cause. It is usually assumed that someone working for a charitable organisation is not primarily motivated by money, as it is common knowledge that charity sector jobs are less well remunerated than those in the private sector. Instead, charity workers appear to be motivated by an ethic of care, shaped by their own particular ethical values, emotional attachments, and political commitments. Many charities specify support for the organisation's aims as a requirement for prospective employees, so in securing their careers, charity workers are assessed not only on their skills, qualifications, or experience but also on their ethics. Indeed, a few of the wildlife centre's employees had been members of the Adopt a Dolphin fund-raising scheme that I describe in chapter 5 as children.

In thinking about charity work and ethical labour, it is instructive to consider it from the other side of the coin, by comparing it with a female-dominated sphere of work that is popularly seen as profit driven, unethical, and even harmful to the self. In her ethnography of London sex workers, Sophie Day describes their strict distinction between their public lives as workers on the one hand and the private realm of home and love on the other. Sex workers were scrupulous in demarcating boundaries that clients, as opposed to partners, could not cross, and many were fastidious about washing and preventing the exchange of bodily fluids with clients, which Day argues is not only about hygiene—with all the assumptions about public and commercial dirt that that implies—but also about maintaining a rigid separation between their outer, public, working self and inner, private, personal self.[17]

Unlike the stigmatised labour of sex workers, charity employees do work that is culturally valued as good, so they benefit from the idea that profession reflects a person's inner self. Whilst sex workers must do a great deal to remove the "taint" of their work, charity professionals are popularly thought of as virtuous and principled. However, the drawback of this association between personal and professional identity is that it is difficult to draw a clear line between work and home life. For those who live in Spey Bay, like Sophie, Willow, and the residential volunteers, this is particularly clear, as they are likely to be called upon whenever something goes wrong, even if they are not officially working that day. So, in fact, charity employees may be exploited—because they feel under pressure to do extra work beyond that for which they are paid or they may hesitate before seeking a pay rise because they do not want to be perceived as being driven by money or because they feel guilty about diverting any of the organisation's resources away from the cause. Unlike sex workers, however, in the popular imagination a young woman working for little or no money caring for turtles on a Caribbean beach is unlikely to be thought of as a victim.

In her discussion of American flight attendants, Hochschild pays attention to the importance that is placed on their appearance by employers, which illustrates the extent to which flight attendants must embody the particular values of their jobs. A young, conventionally attractive, single woman is the ideal because she is thought to be eager to please, wholesome, and compliant whilst also sexually attractive and driven by a sense of fun and adventure. In other words, she will love her job and her behaviour will display this. The logical end point of the "managed heart" of commercialised emotional labour, from the capitalist point of view, is a world in which employees embody their employers' values to such an extent that there is in fact no difference between their personal and professional selves. This is also the ideal of charity work. Whilst charities are by definition not profit driven, like the airline and other private industries, they do prefer that their employees embody their values and that these commitments will have formed prior to their employment, like a natural predisposition.

Recent decades have been characterised by an increasing "feminisation" of the workforce. Ostensibly this term is meant to refer simply to the growing numbers of women taking on paid work outside the home, but with the rise of the service industry and the increasing casualisation of labour, some scholars have pointed out that it also increasingly refers to the "type" of workers favoured by employers, not least because they are cheaper.[18] Cristina Morini argues that the precariousness, mobility, and fragmentation that have come to characterise contemporary working patterns fits with stereotypically feminine characteristics. She also suggests that women are better equipped than men to cope with these situations as they are more used to having insecure positions within the workforce, so existing inequalities are reentrenched.[19] Nina Power has also written about the contradictions of the feminisation of labour and has described how contemporary workers are expected to be "like an advert for yourself,"[20] so that people are always primed for an opportunity, always ready to network and constantly embodying their employability.[21] This is emotional labour, 24/7.

Working for a charity is seen to entail sacrifice, because of the number of low and unpaid jobs it offers, and to be motivated by responsibility, dedication and altruism—all traits that are culturally associated with femininity and domestic labour. The women with paid jobs in the wildlife centre who I have focused on in this chapter—Sophie, Willow, Lauren, Amy, Charlotte, Heather, and Nina—work in these jobs not only because they value the aims of wildlife conservation, but also because they want personally fulfilling careers. Cetacean conservation is the glamorous side of this field and they had all worked in "exotic" locations before coming to Spey Bay. However, the payoff for such fulfilment is a tendency towards low pay (by middle-class standards) and short-term contracts, as well as the competitive nature of the work, which means that many people work as unpaid volunteers and interns for a few years before securing a paid job, which can have knock-on effects on finding a potential partner and having children for men and women. Yet it is a middle-class ideal to find a career that is personally fulfilling and the staff members in the wildlife centre repeatedly told me how, despite the problems and stresses of everyday working life, they felt very fortunate to be paid for doing a job that they loved.[22]

The work of the wildlife centre does not simply reproduce ideologies of femininity—staff members have travelled and moved away from their families for the sake of their careers, their jobs contain elements of "masculine" work including scientific research, public speaking, fund-raising, and campaigning, and they expect to be personally financially independent—but it takes place in a context that relies to a large extent on the successful implementation of a particular ethic that is informed by "feminine" values and in an economic context that puts much of the onus for keeping a job and developing a successful career on the shoulders of the employee. Surrounding charity work with connotations of altruism and compassion offers opportunities for those who participate in it to acquire particular ethical subjectivities, but it also serves to smooth over inequalities in pay and conditions between different sectors of the market, for different working roles, and for workers of different genders.

The ethical labour that staff in the wildlife centre do is not limited to work on themselves, as, whatever their particular job description, they are all to varying extents involved in reproducing the ethical imperative to care for whales, dolphins, and the environment in other people. There is a delicious synchrony to the fact that the particular animals that the people in Spey Bay concern and associate themselves with are whales and dolphins. Not only are they popularly seen as feminine animals, but they are also thought to be caring, sociable, and family oriented and the charity certainly plays on these characteristics in promoting the conservation cause. However, in practice, people's ideas about these animals were a little more complicated. In response to some of the more enthusiastic or anthropomorphic characterisations of cetaceans of people who espoused "hippie" ideas about dolphins and whales, amongst themselves they were keen to demonstrate their awareness of the fact that, whilst there may be similarities between humans and cetaceans, they *are* different species, not least because cetaceans are wild animals.

Quite a few times I heard staff members talking about the fact that pods of dolphins "play" by throwing and catching porpoises. Dolphins do not usually eat porpoises, so this is not hunting or feeding behaviour but is seen instead as a sort of blood sport. They did not mention this in front of visitors or children usually, but on one occasion when I was volunteering with Sophie, a visitor to the centre brought it up whilst he was chatting with us. Sophie responded that the charity that runs the wildlife centre does not deny this behaviour and said, "People tend to see dolphins as these happy, friendly creatures, but they are really wild animals, and we need to remember that." The man agreed and concluded, "A lot of the time, they behave better than humans, anyway." There are periodic accounts in the media of dolphins "saving" humans from danger, such as a case from New Zealand, which was made into a docudrama by BBC2 and shown in February 2008. In this case, some young swimmers were surrounded by a group of bottlenose dolphins, which appeared to be herding them together to protect them from an approaching great white shark. When I mentioned this "altruistic" dolphin case to Sophie whilst on a follow-up trip to Spey Bay after my main period of fieldwork, she dismissed the idea that dolphins could be altruistic out of hand, rolling her eyes and saying firmly, "Yeah, whatever, they're wild animals."

Conclusion

Sophie felt that, with age, she had developed a greater capacity to be responsible for herself and others, suggesting that she was more mature and less "selfish." This indicates what she feels are the important qualities for mothering. It also implies both a sense of agency and a feeling that the desire, and ability, to become a parent came inevitably with age. It furthermore suggests that learning to care for others is part of becoming a mature adult.[23] The concept of the stable environment encapsulates the ideals of parenthood, but it also implies a sense that some things just happen naturally, or in other words, that there is a realm of human experience that lies beyond our capacity for making individual choices or shaping our own destinies. As the word "stable" suggests, it is about achieving a balance between responsible planning and ethical ideals on the one hand and biological drives and natural dispositions on the other; it is a process of making biology fit with parental ethics—and vice versa.

In the epigraph to this chapter, Arlie Hochschild writes about a "natural preserve of feeling, a place to be kept 'forever wild,'" which she suggests is becoming "scarce."[24] This epigraph captures some of the congruities between ideas of the natural on both the individual and the environmental scales that are at play here. Both the idea of the unmanaged heart and the notion of wild nature suggest a counterpoint to human activity and, perhaps, the tyranny of choice. If, ultimately, we are all "hemmed in by biology," as Willow put it, then perhaps there are a number of different "right" times to have a child or "good" ways to parent, as long as they are all natural.

The idea of the unmanaged heart, of natural feeling or wild emotion, is one that emerges alongside capitalism; it is the counterpoint to the professional self whose contours are formed and processed through the habitus of work. But, as Hochschild points out, even emotions can be professionalised and commodified, and as I have suggested here, so can ethics. To be clear, I am not arguing that charity work is simply a sop to capitalist hegemony, but I am suggesting that it takes place in a context in which the reach of capitalism is fathoms deep. The ethical labour of people in Spey Bay is a recognition of and a response to political and economic structures and values that seem to put profit above the well-being and stability of the environment. It resists the idea that greed and selfishness are necessarily the main drivers of human nature, whilst recognising that money and work are vitally interconnected and that self-interest is implicated in any ethical decision.

// Beginnings

Scotland has always been part of my origin story, though I never lived there before my fieldwork. My father is Scottish and my parents met as a consequence of both studying at St. Andrews University. When they divorced, whilst I was a baby, my father moved up to Edinburgh. I made regular trips to see him and, later, my stepmother, half sister, and half brother during the school holidays whilst I was growing up. He would often take us to see the sights of Scotland, its landscape of villages, castles, forests, and mountains. The Scott Monument, Culzean castle, the pretty painted houses of Tobermory, ham sandwiches and fruit cake eaten in the back of the car, the music of The Corries, the smell of the Caledonian brewery hanging over western Edinburgh (sometimes sweet and malty, sometimes strangely akin to cat food), the train through to Glasgow, the small glass of (Dow's) port I was allowed at Hogmanay—this was the Scotland that was part of my childhood and I took it with me when I went to do fieldwork.

I had thought, naively, that my own Scottish roots might bring me some kudos as a sort of returned native, but I was largely wrong. Most people I met weren't that interested in knowing others' origins, preferring to take them at face value, in the present tense. Anyway, my region-less middle-class English accent and reluctance to adopt full-time outdoor wear were probably difficult to overlook despite the evidence of my surname, my ability to understand Aberdonian accents, and my extensive knowledge of Historic Scotland sites.

My beginnings add up to an inevitable interest in kinship and reproduction. Let me explain by offering one slice of the cake, a bit of context to my own take on reproductive ethics. My dad was adopted as a baby and knew nothing about it until he reached adulthood. He only started to find out about his mother, grandparents, uncles, and cousins after his half sister appeared in his life when he was in his mid-forties. With his adoptive parents dead and this new origin story emerging, he began the process of excavating and remaking his identity. His birth mother, who had never married, had died decades earlier, giving birth to twins. All three were found in her tenement flat in Dundee two weeks later by her father, my great-grandfather, the owner of a local bakery, who had just returned from a business trip.

It was only in 2011 that we discovered there were two more half sisters, alive and well and, it turned out, keen to meet their new/old relatives. My dad, the eldest, and each of his half sisters had been adopted at birth, in different cities and by different couples, who probably didn't know there were siblings out there. The sisters share a father, who was married to someone else and had more children with his wife and another woman besides. We can only surmise, from holiday snaps, that my dad's father was a Glaswegian bus driver who drove his mother on a European coach tour the year before my dad was born. My dad is the spitting image of that coach driver. No one knows why my grandmother kept getting pregnant and why each time she was compelled to give the child up for adoption.[1] No one knows if that was also her intention for the twins she carried last.

The process of discovering these new kin has also been one of amassing coincidences along the way—one of my aunts has the same name as my sister and lives just around the corner from where my partner grew up, another has the same model and colour of car as my dad and people see physical resemblances everywhere, especially between my aunts and me (despite the fact that I have always been told that I look like my mother). It was therefore not a complete surprise when I received the news from my dad in 2013 that they had tracked down his latest long-lost sister to Lossiemouth, just a twenty-minute drive west of Spey Bay. When I finally met her in 2014, it turned out she was a regular visitor to the wildlife centre and we speculated about whether we had ever met before without realising it.

Future Generations

It is a little late to be saying that man should not
interfere with nature or try to help it on a little.
. . . In any case, the problem is different now;
nature needs our help if it is to survive what has
already been done to it.

—*Lord Flowers, Human Fertilisation and Embryology
Bill debate, House of Lords, 7 December 1989*

The Biological Clock

Six months after we had celebrated her birthday in a pizza
restaurant, Charlotte asked me if I had come across anyone who
was infertile because of polycystic ovary syndrome (PCOS). We
were standing outside her back door in the biting January cold,
whilst her partner, Mark, watched football on the television
inside with Steve and Chris. Charlotte had arrived in Moray
shortly before I did and we had quickly become good friends
after I started volunteering in the wildlife centre. When I first
met her, she seemed quite sure that she and Mark, who was
in the RAF, would have a child within the next few years. Although money was tight for them and Mark was facing service in Iraq, she believed that because they loved each other and
wanted to spend their lives together they would make it work.

That night, as the men settled into the football, Charlotte
had taken me aside, explaining that she wanted to talk to me
"in a professional capacity." She told me that she was due to see
her doctor the next day about some menstrual problems she had
been experiencing. She was worried that she might have PCOS.

I reminded her that I was not medically trained but talked it through with her and tried to reassure her that even if it did turn out to be PCOS it did not necessarily mean she would be unable to have children. I felt uneasy about Charlotte's perception of my "professional" expertise. I had, of course, explained my research project to her when we first became acquainted, as I did with everyone I met during fieldwork, but I was concerned about how she understood it and how I could make it clearer. I believe now that Charlotte turned to me for a "professional" view in the absence of anyone with any better expertise. I was always careful not to express any strong views about infertility or ART during my fieldwork, so I think she saw me as an interested and nonjudgemental person to turn to, to discuss these issues, but my discomfort at being treated as an expert certainly reminded me of my ethical responsibilities towards her and all of my "informants."

That night, Charlotte told me that she had always been unsure as to whether she wanted children and now she felt she was in some way paying for that uncertainty. She said, "It's like I've said I don't want children too many times and now someone's said, 'ok,' and now the door might have been shut, I want to have them." After a long medical investigation, she was diagnosed with some benign ovarian cysts as well as endometriosis. Halfway through this investigation, she suffered a new problem, when Mark left her. She moved out of the house where they were cohabiting and into her colleague Amy's tiny spare bedroom. Although she was not in the least self-pitying about Mark's departure, Charlotte often discussed with me what she was going to do now that she was single and eventually decided to move back to England to retrain for a new career.

A few months after the breakup, Charlotte had to have a laparoscopy. I drove her to the hospital and stayed with her for two nights as she recovered from the surgery. I got a sense from talking to her around that time that, whilst before she had been concerned about her fertility in relation to her gynaecological issues, the breakup had made the question of whether she might be infertile a little less pressing because she assumed that she would not, and ideally should not, become a parent unless she was in a stable relationship. A few months after the laparoscopy, when she was getting ready to move back to England, Charlotte talked with me about the reproductive schedule that she and Mark had once set for themselves, recalling that they had planned to start having children within the next three years. This led her to reflect on her new circumstances: "If I met somebody really quickly it might still be the plan for the next three years, but then comes the scary thought, what if there isn't [anyone]? What if I haven't met anyone by the time I'm thirty? What do I do?"

When Charlotte's fertility was called into question and she found herself without a partner, she experienced a rupture in her planned life course,[1] which led her to consider herself, her former partner, her relationships with others, and her future in a new light. Charlotte had, as she said herself, always been somewhat ambivalent about becoming a parent. Before she met Mark, she had been engaged to a man she went to school with but broke it off after spending her first year at university and realising that, as she put it, "there's more to life than getting married, having a family, and settling down." After moving back to London after fieldwork, I invited Charlotte to dinner one night so we could catch up. We talked about her health, her future plans, and the course she had just started. Her expectations for parenthood came up in the conversation and she reflected that she would only like to have a child if she not only had the right partner but also a stable career. As she put it, "I definitely want to have both."

As Charlotte's experience demonstrates, ideas about reproduction model the making not only of people but also of the future.[2] Charlotte's potential infertility affected her in various ways—it caused her painful, inconvenient, and embarrassing physical symptoms, it put her under pressure to make important decisions before she was ready to, it made her more aware of the contingency of reproductive choice and biological control, and it forced her to think about the future, all at a time when the foundations of the good life she had been making had been pulled out from under her.

Charlotte's story illustrates the salient connections between fertility, reproduction, and visions of the future, even when an individual is ambivalent about whether she wants to have children at all. From Charlotte's point of view, remaining agnostic about whether she would pursue the project of having children one day was never really an option. As I mentioned in the last chapter, Charlotte was not the only woman who referred to her age when discussing her reproductive aspirations with me, and there seemed to be tacit agreement amongst women in Spey Bay that thirty was the magic age at which they should have a good idea of their reproductive future. This makes the significance of timing and choice, and the linked sense that there are "natural limits" on women's reproductive capacities, clear. In this chapter, I will develop these points by discussing the wider importance of time and visions of the future in reproduction, particularly in relation to people's anxieties about the long-term effects of technological intervention in human reproduction.

There is a strain of environmentalist discourse that emphasises the importance of stabilising the human population in creating an environmentally sustainable future, though most campaigners are careful to emphasise that they are aspiring to facilitate reproductive choice rather than encouraging eugenicist population control. Some people in Spey Bay are interested in how an increasing human population will impact the planet and natural resources, but this was not a common topic of conversation. They did not assume that there was a simple line of cause and effect between human activity and environmental degradation, though they did see links between reproduction and the (in)stability of the environment, which goes with a more general assumption that we should consider the environment in every action and decision we take. This chapter explores how ideas about the environment and the state of the natural world are implicated in reproductive decision making for people in

Spey Bay and how they think human reproduction—especially technologically assisted reproduction—might affect the environment in the future.

An Endangered Future

In the previous chapter, I introduced Erin's concept of the stable environment. As her use of the word "environment" indicates, this is a multilayered phenomenon that encompasses the biological, relational, social, economic, and ecological worlds and it can variously and even simultaneously mean a pregnant woman's body, the family home, the natural landscape, the planet, and various other "environments" in between. In talking about reproduction and reproductive decision making, people in Spey Bay made connections between these worlds, indicating their sense of the natural fit between them and of the ramifications of decisions across them. In thinking about the future of human reproduction, people did not worry only about their own children or grandchildren but also about unknown and as yet unborn future generations, including those of other species.

People in Spey Bay did not dwell on the past and tended to locate (potential) crisis in the future. They did have some anxieties about the present, but they did not express deep concern about crumbling social mores and their political attitudes were generally left-of-centre or left-wing. Ostensibly the locus of their anxieties was not in the social world but in the natural one, though of course these cannot be entirely disentangled, as they also placed the responsibility for climate change and environmental degradation on people. As might be expected for people involved in conservation, much of their concern about the future focused on endangerment. As Timothy Choy says in his ethnography of Hong Kong environmentalism, the idea of endangerment parcels up the past, present, and future, implying a need to insulate each from the other, and he describes endangerment as provoking "anticipatory nostalgia." He says:

To speak of an endangered species is to speak of a form of life that threatens to become extinct in the near future; it is to raise the stakes in a controversy so that certain actions carry the consequences of destroying the possibility of life's continued existence. Species can be endangered, as can ecosystems. And, as environmentalists grapple increasingly with the tight bonds that can be formed between people and places, between situated practices and specific landscapes, and between what are commonly glossed as culture and nature, discourses of endangerment have come to structure not only narrowly construed environmental politics, but also politics of cultural survival.[3]

In Spey Bay, people are concerned about the future of the natural world and about species survival, and they celebrate a sense of "community" where they live. At a surface level, then, it might seem that they are attempting to re-create a halcyon past in a rural idyll, but this is not really an accurate rendering of life there. For example, the people I knew in Spey Bay did not lament the decline of the fishing industry like the people in Lancashire described by Jeanette Edwards in *Born and Bred* mourn the loss of the slipper factories,[4] not only because many of them do not have family members who depended on that industry for their livelihoods but also because it is seen as partially culpable for the present and future dangers that the natural world is facing. Rather than bemoaning a general decline in "community values" or "tradition," they see the fact that places like Moray offer a sense of warmth and belonging as a sign of hope. But whilst present life in Spey Bay is not characterised by nostalgia for a lost, better past, the people who live there do fear being nostalgic for what they have in the present when they reach the future. And as I talked to people about technological treatments for infertility, it became clear that their fears of future endangerment were not confined to marine mammals but extended to their own species.

Scotland has the lowest birthrate of the nations that make up the UK and is below "replacement rate" (i.e., fewer than two children per couple), though this is currently balanced out by migration.[5] In my interviews and conversations with people in Spey Bay, it became apparent that many were aware of Scotland's low fertility. Like most governments, the Scottish Government does not have a formal fertility policy, but it does recognise that the provision of statutory child care, maternity leave, and fiscal benefits can influence people's decisions.[6] In 2013, the Scottish Government announced additional funding to end the "postcode lottery" of access to NHS fertility treatment in Scotland,[7] with the aim of reducing waiting times to twelve months by 2015. Under the new regime, eligible patients can have two full cycles of IVF treatment and unlimited frozen embryo transfers up to the recipient's fortieth birthday. Those who live in the NHS Grampian region, which covers Moray, have historically been the main losers in this postcode lottery. For example, the Scottish Executive, as it was then called, reported that the average waiting time for IVF on the NHS for eligible couples in Grampian was sixty months in 2005, which was an increase from twenty-four months just four years earlier and by far the longest waiting time in Scotland in that period.[8]

When I was interviewing them, I asked people in Spey Bay about whether they thought the state should have any role in encouraging a particular birthrate in Scotland or whether it should offer incentives for people to have children whilst they are younger, though this was also the sort of topic that came up in general conversation from time to time. Generally people were uncomfortable with the state intervening in people's reproductive decision making and felt that, given the relatively dense population in the UK as a whole, increasing the birthrate in Scotland was not a primary concern. Indeed, the relative lack of people and consequent areas of comparative wilderness are part of what makes Moray "beautiful." They were also quite positive about immigration to Scotland and felt that foreign migrants, including especially the then quite recent influx of Eastern European migrants following the accession of Poland and other countries to the European Union in 2004, were beneficial to the country as a whole. People perceived infertility as a physiological condition with negative emotional effects that might be treated medically and so thought it fair and humane to provide access to fertility treatments wherever possible, but some voiced doubts about whether the NHS should allocate much money to this type of treatment given its finite resources. Whilst they were sympathetic to the infertile and the "natural" desire to have biogenetically related children, no one thought that having children is a right.

People in Spey Bay perceived that the increasing interest of women in building their own careers was leading to both lower birthrates and a trend towards women having children later in life. In relaying her own plans for future parenthood (see previous chapter), Lauren suggested to me, though she immediately corrected herself, that contraception had been "forced down our throats" and that having taken the Pill might make it harder to get pregnant when she decided she was ready to have children and stopped taking it. There is evidence that, after discontinuing the Pill, women's bodies can take a few months to return to normal fertility, but this is typically temporary and is comparable to the effects of other forms of contraception.[9] Lauren, like many other people who worked as paid staff members in the wildlife centre, has a university degree in the natural sciences and her particular job is concerned with science communication. Her vivid statement about birth control suggests both her sense of personal responsibility for choosing the "right" time to get pregnant and a wider ambivalence about technological interventions in life itself.[10]

Charlotte, who had previously worked as a pharmacist, told me that she was uncomfortable with the fact that her doctor had prescribed the contraceptive pill to help manage the symptoms of her endometriosis. She felt, based on previous experience of taking it, that the Pill was not compatible with her body and told me, "My body doesn't want to be on the Pill." Both her and Lauren's comments suggest their complex and ambivalent feelings about the fact that they can (attempt to) control their reproductive systems through technology. Whilst Lauren had not, as far as I know, suffered any of the medical problems that Charlotte was experiencing at this time, they shared a keen sense of reproductive risk, in terms of a heightened awareness that conception is not necessarily inevitable, as well as a sense that too much control over biology may have unintended consequences. These fears point to their, and their friends', wider fears about an endangered future, for humans and for the environment.

In interviews, I asked people whether they thought that rates of infertility were related to the ways in which people live their lives. When I had conceived this question I had anticipated that people might criticise "lifestyle choices," but whilst some did reflect on societal change in this way, many also drew connections between human reproduction, the natural world, and future crisis, and in quite disparate ways. For example, Jenny, a social worker with two adult children, was prompted to think of the interaction between human actions, biology, and the environment, suggesting that oestrogens in the water supply were contributing to a "feminisation of men," and others talked of pollutants causing fish to "change sex." Over the last decade or so, there has been a steady drip of news stories about the potential effects of natural and synthetic chemicals in water supplies on humans and wildlife, which Jenny was alluding to. Researchers have tended to focus on the effects of chemicals from plastic containers and packaging, detergents, food, and cosmetics,[11] whilst some anti-contraception campaigners have asserted that oral contraceptives are causing environmental damage, though the scientific evidence suggests that oral contraceptives are not a primary cause of oestrogenic compounds in water.[12]

Public knowledge about both reproduction and the environment is coloured by the intense passions of competing interest groups, which have often been reflected in hesitant or sensationalist media reporting, but stories of chemicals in waterways

"causing" fish to change sex have captured the attention of journalists and campaigners. Various scholars have written about
the environmentalist movement's framing of pollutants, including the endocrine disrupting chemicals (EDCs) that Jenny referred to.[13] Whilst environmentalism is a very broad church, it
is worth noting the way that gender is made through activism
on this exemplary issue. In discussing the way in which EDCs
and similar pollutants cross and disturb boundaries of time,
space, gender, generation, and species, Celia Roberts critiques
the heteronormativity deployed by many environmental activists
including big-hitters like Greenpeace, the World Wide Fund for
Nature, and Friends of the Earth in getting across their concerns about the ecological and biological—but also, implicitly,
social—effects of toxic substances on living populations. Roberts
points out that "rather than using the current moment of crisis
in human-animal-environment interimplications to expose the
assumption of 'natural' relationships between these categories,
environmentalist, mass media and popular science discourses
of endocrine disruptors . . . reproduce heteronormative figurations of both hormones and sex/gender."[14] These campaigns are
effective—and interesting to journalists—because they touch
on existing assumptions about our future existence relying on
"normal" sexual reproduction, pervasive fears about runaway
scientific progress, the universality of maternal responsibility,
and the sense that future generations will inherit the consequences of previous ones' choices and actions.

Responding to the same question that I had asked Jenny,
Sophie was reminded of what she had learned about animal
husbandry as an undergraduate student. She said:

> When I was at university we had a couple of classes which
> talked about fertility and we were talking about farm ani
> mals, the lecturer was then just bringing into play that ac
> tually humans are pretty crap at being fertile if you com
> pare them to the farm animals and the fact that we breed
> those over the successive generations to be really fertile. And

because there are maybe some things that don't naturally select out because people who can have some help to allow fertility—maybe there is an element of that, that they're all going a bit down the scientific route. So I'd be a bit averse to . . . go down the line that says, "Oh well, we've almost asked for it," but I do think that there are some things that we can't get away from, that probably we are going to find it harder and harder [to reproduce]. Then again, I suppose . . . from the ecologist's point of view, I might say, "Well, there's quite a lot of humans and maybe this is just the way it goes, maybe this is the way the cycle goes."

I will return to Sophie's thoughts on the connections between fertility, biology, agriculture, and ecology and the way she slips between different models of time later in the chapter. Her specific concern about the rising human population, which is, as I mentioned earlier, a common feature of environmentalist discourse, also came up in discussions about adoption with others. People generally thought that adoption was a morally and socially responsible option for childless couples but that wanting to have a child "of your own" was understandable and that the realities of adoption in the UK were onerous and unsatisfactory. None had adopted children themselves, though some who did not have children said that they would consider doing so. In discussions about adoption, one of the ideas I heard frequently was that there are a number of children "out there," and as Willow put it, "it would be nice in an ideal world if people would look after the children we already have."

Andrew, a residential volunteer in the wildlife centre, echoed Sophie's concerns about what the biological and demographic consequences of assisted conception might be. He said that, now that infertile people can "conceive with science," "we've evolved beyond evolution." He went on to reflect on how increasing access to ART might affect the environment more generally: "There's huge pressure on this planet in terms of resources for a number of people and so one part of me says, if you can't do it

naturally, you shouldn't do it at all. On the other hand, I can totally, entirely understand on an individual level that if you want
a kid then you're gonna do everything that you can possibly do
to have that child."

Natural Limits

Sarah Franklin has identified an intellectual lineage of anxiety about technology being coupled with fears about the future
of reproduction that goes back to (at least) Plato.[15] In *Phaedrus*,
Plato decried writing as a shabby imitation of verbal rhetoric
and Socrates added that writing is a sterile act that produces
only barren fruit.[16] As Franklin puts it, in this dialogue, "the
artifice of written inscription is equated with a loss of humanity,
a loss of truth, and a loss of self."[17] Franklin applies this concern
about the technology of writing to the more recent technology
of IVF to consider what it is to be "after IVF," in an echo of
Strathern's[18] exposition of what it means to be "after nature." As
Franklin says, the ancient example of Plato's and Socrates' mis-
trust of writing, as a controversial reproductive technology of
their time, shows the ambivalence that technology provokes and
how vital ideas about time, progress, kinship, and inheritance
are to that ambivalence.

Ambivalence about technology parallels ambivalence about
the future. "It is the fear of degeneration in the wake of technological change, set against a more confident expectation of
an improved, more fruitful, future, that has long characterized
technological ambivalence," Franklin writes.[19] But, as she continues, one of the most striking characteristics of these fears is
how quickly they turn to questions about the future of kinship
and fertility. It may seem obvious that ART would provoke concerns about kinship, since it has been supposed that this is what
they are all about, but Franklin makes the important point that
in fact this relationship between technology and kinship has
not historically been confined to ART—it may even apply to

something as (now) banal and authoritative as writing. Similarly, when people worry about the future of kinship and reproduction, they may be talking about much more than family.

People in Spey Bay were generally nuanced in their reproductive ethics, but there were examples of ART that we talked about which provoked strong negative reactions, specifically those which seemed to be the result of (potential) parents putting their own needs above those of their children. Practices like postmenopausal women using IVF and the creation of "designer babies" were most problematic, as they seemed to represent an excess of individual choice that could both denature reproduction and dehumanise kinship. Embedded in people's ideas about the future of human reproduction are their judgements about the limits of nature and the responsibilities that people have towards protecting it.

Joanna was strongly in favour of allowing people access to ART through the NHS, but she drew the line at "designer babies."[20] She said that if parents use ART because they "want to make their child a perfect child, then, no [they shouldn't be allowed to], because *that's not having children*. If you have a child, then that's your child to bring up, no matter what they look like" (emphasis added). Nina had a similar view. She said she would "draw the line at people getting picky," such as foetal sex selection or the creation of "designer babies," explaining that "it's just playing god, really, and I don't think it's right. I think you should be satisfied with what you get and I think giving [parents] the gift of a child should be enough. . . . I mean, if they can't have children, fine, give them help, but then don't start messing with nature more than you already have done."

Jenny's partner, Paul, who was also born in England, is a mature student and local volunteer in the wildlife centre. His own father was in his mid-forties when he was born and he thought that women using ART when they have passed menopause was "a bit selfish." He said, "I don't think it's fair on children, really. And it's so unnatural. I don't know if we should as a human race be necessarily moving—I feel this about a lot of things—I don't think we should necessarily be moving away from nature all the time into some world of science. It just seems the wrong way."

Like Paul, Lauren was very concerned about the prospect of postmenopausal women using ART:

> I don't really like that medical science is pushing us beyond natural human boundaries, as far as it is. . . . To some extent, there have to be some lines [where] you let nature take its course, and, you know, as hard as it is for the woman who doesn't want, choose to have a child 'til she's fifty, there are some natural limits there and there are kind of reasons why your body doesn't want you to have a child when you're fifty, and that partially is because you'll be sixty-five when your child's fifteen and, you know, you are pushing those situations. The sticky point [is] that men can still conceive at that point in time, . . . I hate to say it but that's the way it is, is how I think I feel and I think that I quite like that there are some things, I suppose that are just, "that's the way it is." . . . I'm sure in a lot of cases, these are very educated people, but you know, there should be some choices where money can't buy a different reality.

Sophie agreed with Lauren and Paul but had reservations about the political correctness of her judgement. When I interviewed her, she told me, "Personally, although it goes right against some of my right-on views, I think that [no longer being able to conceive after menopause] *is* nature, and—unless this is some medical condition which has meant that menopause has come in way earlier in life—if it's natural, no, I don't think there should be any intervention then, especially when there are kids who need homes and all those things. But that's quite a personal view" (original emphasis). When I was chatting with Sophie the next day, she told me that she had been feeling some remorse about making such a strong judgement. It seemed that she had surprised herself by being so forthright and by going against her usually "right-on views," yet she did not retract what she had said. The prospect of an older woman using ART to have a child because she was too old to conceive "naturally" caused her to pit her politics against her sense of the natural and the latter won out.

James Laidlaw has written about the importance of retaining space for "freedom" in anthropological descriptions of ethics.[21] For Laidlaw, drawing on Foucault,[22] when a subject steps back and reflects on different ways of acting or responds to dilemmas, this is an act of freedom. He therefore argues that freedom is intrinsic to ethical reflection and the crafting of the self as an ethical subject. Michael Lambek, whose discomfort with the rhetorical baggage of "freedom" I share, has argued that such acts are better described as judgements.[23] Although I am loath to add yet another suggestion to theirs, I do find both "freedom" and "judgement" problematic terms given their rhetorical associations. Instead, I see this kind of reflective action as an intrinsic part of ethical labour. Whatever the preferred nomenclature, though, I agree with both Laidlaw and Lambek that fashioning oneself as an ethical subject is not about unthinkingly following moral strictures but exercising the capacity to reflect upon the decisions, judgements, and actions one takes. In reflecting upon the ethics of postmenopausal women using assisted conception to conceive, Sophie (self-)consciously balanced her apprehension of natural ethics against the "right-on" ethic of embracing diversity and questioning conventionality. She thus demonstrated Laidlaw's point that attempting to identify the distinctive moral system of a particular group of people will not allow one to adequately capture how people make ethical choices or lead ethical lives.[24] As Joel Robbins says, "Ethnographies of ethics need to attend not only to the socially given aspects of particular subject positions, but also to the idiosyncrasies inhabitants of them develop as part of their ethical work on themselves."[25] What Sophie's dilemma between politics and nature also demonstrates is the way that reproductive technologies make our assumptions about the workings of kinship, biology, and gender explicit. For Sophie, in this particular case, nature provided the ethical scaffolding for her view of what was the right time and means by which to become a parent.

Time

In her comments comparing the fertility of farm animals with that of humans, which was something she had learned about in the past and brought with her to the present, Sophie switched between different models of time. The timeline of animal breeding, which she overlapped with Darwinian evolutionary time, is a linear one in which traits such as high fertility can be bred in. In this model, future generations are a product of the choices and actions of previous ones, which can be progressive or degenerative depending on what is bred in. In thinking about the distant future, though, Sophie referred to "the ecologist's point of view," which is cyclical. By referring to ecological time, Sophie was making not only her concerns about technological hubris and poor husbandry leading to human endangerment clear but also her sense that humans are only one part of the environment. What Sophie's example also demonstrates is that the environment plays a part in reproduction and fertility but that modes of reproduction also affect the environment; reproduction and environment rely upon each other for stability.

As these examples show, people used images of movement and momentum when they described their concerns about the future, linking space and time as they outlined their fears about human activity becoming divorced from nature through scientific overreaching. It is well established that science and technology are, in Western thinking at least, closely associated with progress and forward movement and much of the positive rhetoric—and marketing—surrounding ART promotes its promissory value. This resonates with the popular idea that children are their parents' future. Like space, how we envisage time is closely linked with how we see our environments and with our visions of the future. But progressive linear teleologies are not the only models of time that make sense to people.

Phil Macnaghten and John Urry write that whilst modernity was associated with clock time, along with the goals of mastery over nature and industrialised work patterns, the contemporary age is characterised by two further experiences of time as simultaneously imperceptibly fast, "instantaneous time" and unimaginably slow, "glacial time."[26] Glacial time is associated with environmentalist conceptions of the world, which also posit a planetary conception of space and appeals to a global citizenship. A sense of time as glacial and culture as global is necessary, Macnaghten and Urry argue, to compel people to act in favour of the environment.[27] As such, the environment is no longer an "other" waiting to be mastered but an intrinsic part of human experience. This has various effects including reinforcing the sense that environmental disasters affect us all, including future generations. It also promotes greater fluidity in individuals' and communities' attachments to place. This fits with people in Spey Bay's sense that they are part of the natural world and with their efforts to build good lives that value the present and future connections between people, animals, and place.

Franklin has pointed out the importance of time in building public support for ART in the UK through the example of the establishment in law of the fourteen-day limit on human embryo research based on the emergence of the "primitive streak," which neatly ties together biological and legal time. As she says, "Biological development is a useful idiom precisely because of the extent to which it can be seen as a non-specific discourse of temporality, existing in a realm that is both supra-legal and scientifically verifiable."[28] She also describes how the apparently natural and universal timelines of human life and development have become fused with ideas about the future lives and health of the human population, so that medical technologies that "assist" them appear to be following logical, progressive trajectories.[29]

In the concerns about breaching "natural limits" that people in Spey Bay expressed to me, they were not simply reproducing a teleological view of history. Andrew even suggested that ART had caused humans to "evolve beyond evolution," which is a rather cataclysmic idea. The future, in their view, is the product of choices and activities, though these are never fully predictable or "rational" but are contingent on context and relations. As the species with the greatest power to spoil our environment, humans, they believe, have a particular duty to try to prevent catastrophic destruction by responsible and careful planning.

In *After Nature*, Marilyn Strathern explored British people's sense in the late twentieth-century "epoch" that with the rise of biotechnology, fears about environmental crisis and changes in family constitutions nature would no longer seem capable of acting as a fundamental grounding for human activity.[30] ART and the effects of human industry on the environment both created a sense, she argued, that there is "less" nature in the world. Strathern's crucial claim about this epoch, when ART was new and the Green movement was still at the fringes of public debate, was that with increasingly minute manipulations of biology and the natural world through science and technology, nature's "grounding function" would come to "disappear"; its capacity to act as an ultimate reference point would become destabilised. With this, she wrote, "[nature] no longer provides a model or analogy for the very idea of context. With the destabilising of relation, context and grounding, it is no surprise that the present crisis (epoch) appears an ecological one. We are challenged to imagine neither intrinsic forms nor self-regulating systems."[31]

Strathern's predictions in *After Nature* were provocations—by portraying a future in which nature would lose its grounding function, she was not only outlining the profound consequences that ART might have on the way British people think about kinship, society, nature, and knowledge but also implying that nature might in fact weather the storm. As Franklin says, there is a "rolling process" of naturalisation and denaturalisation in people's ideas about reproduction.[32] Sands may shift, but nature is tenacious. Its conceptual force continues to haunt both ethnography and anthropological theory, despite our declarations that it is no less "cultural" than anything else. One reason for this is its polysemy, its ability to alter its shape and scale.[33] Nature is both context and fact, external and intrinsic, environment and entity. In thinking about infertility and ART, people in Spey Bay typically turned to nature as a source of ethical guidance; in nature, they found fertile grounds for their sense of what was good.

Conclusion

The idea of "natural limits" in reproduction demonstrates the tension that people in Spey Bay felt between being nonjudgemental of others' personal lives and respectful of individuals' autonomy whilst also protecting the integrity of nature, which is a familiar dilemma for people involved in the environmental movement. The concept of natural limits suggests that they believe that nature has a breaking point and that problems with fertility are a sign that nature is reaching this point. Whilst people sympathised with the desire to have biogenetically related children and supported individuals' rights to access medical treatment, they feared that outsourcing parts of the reproductive process to third parties or petri dishes could breed in infertility in the long term. Like the technological ambivalence expressed by Plato in relation to writing, they were concerned that the hubristic use of science and technology might cause humans to become an endangered species in the future. These concerns pose the question of whether there are some natural limits that human technology cannot overcome.

People in Spey Bay see whales and dolphins as victims of human choices manifested in industrial pollution, the erstwhile whaling industry, current large-scale fishing practices, and the overproduction of carbon emissions that cause climate change. They also worry that humans might create a potentially bleak future for ourselves by attempting to control our reproduction through technology rather than "letting nature take its course."

These fears reflect concerns about runaway scientific "progress" and about the limits of human biology, but they also point to ambivalence about choice and human nature. The interconnections people made between different lively environments demonstrate the tension between human choice and activity on the one hand and the givens of nature and biology on the other. It should be evident that this is not a rigid dichotomy, which is precisely why it is experienced as tense.

In the coming chapters, the importance of an ethic of responsibility—towards kin, friends, environment, and community—will become increasingly apparent. People in Spey Bay demonstrate responsibility by using contraception to prevent pregnancy at the "wrong" time and by doing what they can to build fulfilling and stable lives for future generations. They do "good" work that demonstrates their commitment to caring for the environment, and they try to earn and spend money in "ethical" ways. Building a stable environment entails making choices, which are always contingent rather than absolute. People do not see immanent power in money, science, or technology but place responsibility for the future squarely at the feet of people and the choices they make. But, it is important to note, in identifying the motives that drive reproductive decisions, they ponder the effects of those decisions, not only on that particular family but also on their wider community, the natural world, and future generations. Their concerns about the future reflect the necessity of ethical limits and nature's capacity for providing guidance in discerning those limits. But, as the next two chapters will show, nature has not just an ethical potency but also a normative force.

// *The Water of Life*

A number of my friends, as well as my parents and siblings, visited me during fieldwork. When they came, it was a good opportunity to press pause and realise what novel assumptions had flowed into my quotidian thinking.

Apart from salmon, whisky is what puts the Spey valley on the map, so I would often take people to distilleries. It seemed a quintessentially Scottish thing to do. Although many other countries make whisky, malt whisky made in Scotland still has a particular cachet. According to a briefing for the Scottish Parliament by the Scotch Whisky Association, whisky brings £4 billion a year in gross value to the economy and supports 35,000 Scottish jobs; it also brings £3.45 billion in exports and is Scotland's second largest export after oil and gas.[1]

The Spey valley has the highest concentration of whisky distilleries in Scotland. Many are open to the public, and tourists and whisky enthusiasts can enjoy tours of the distilleries with an overview of the distilling process, from the sourcing of the ingredients to the long maturation of the spirit towards graduation as a legally certifiable Scottish malt whisky—a minimum of three years and one day. These tours are popular with tourists, not least because it is customary for them to end with an opportunity to taste a dram of the whisky made in that distillery. Most tours were, at the time, free, though visitors were enthusiastically pointed in the direction of the gift shop, where a range of whiskies and whisky-based products were available to purchase.

There is something in the popular view of Scottish malt whisky that seems to fit with the landscape, as if this "water of life" springs up organically from the very soil. In a way, it does. Whisky is made, as anyone who has visited a distillery will know, from three ingredients: grain, water, and yeast. Distilleries not only are the complex of buildings that house the mash tuns, washbacks, spirit safes, casks, and warehouses that make whisky but also include natural springs that provide the water and often their own barley fields too. The provenance of the yeast is usually an industrial secret. There is even some speculation that whisky picks up some of its flavour from the air around it whilst it is maturing. It is no coincidence, then, that whiskies usually have the same name as their distilleries, which are themselves often named after the settlements in which they are located. Even though each whisky gets much of its distinctive flavour from the recycled sherry, bourbon, or wine casks in which it is aged and some whiskies are coloured with the caramel dye E150a, the landscape in which it is made and matured is an important part of its constitution. In the world of Scottish malt whisky, place is more than provenance—it is embodied in the very product and ingested by the consumer.

Although I never heard the word *terroir* used in conjunction with whisky, there is surely a very similar idea at work here.[2] No doubt many of the visitors to Scottish distilleries, when they get home and open the bottle of whisky they bought in the distillery gift shop, are taken back by that honeyed, oaky smell to the neat green lawns, trickling spring, and purple-brown mountains of the place in which it originated. But whilst nostalgia is important in the marketing of whisky, whisky-making is in itself a future-oriented craft, since the longer it is matured, the "better" it will taste; it relies on future generations to care for the environment in which it is made for its increasing gustatory and economic value.

The distillery to which I took visitors most often was Glenfiddich. Owned by William Grant & Sons, it is located at the heart of the Spey valley and tour guides emphasise the "purity" of the adjacent Robbie Dhu spring, where they source the water for their whisky. As befits the best-selling Scotch in the world, with a recent annual turnover of £1 billion,[3] Glenfiddich offers a slick—some might even say camp—visitor experience. Even the visitor toilets are a suite of wood-panelled rooms with a large open fireplace and stag antler candelabra. On my first trip there, I took a visiting friend from London who had once worked as a market researcher. He described Glenfiddich distillery as "a corporate wet dream," a description I found amusing but a little jarring. What version of Scotland was I unwittingly presenting to him and how could I reconcile it with the Scotland I encountered every day? At Glenfiddich, my latest Scotland, the one of impromptu get-togethers over vegetarian fajitas, battles with "humane" mouse traps, habitual fleece-wearing, and evenings spent discussing the (de)merits of utopian community projects over inexpensive Fairtrade wine, was like another country.

Before the distillery tour begins, visitors are ushered into a purpose-built cinema to watch a ten-minute film about the history of Glenfiddich, which opened its distillery on Christmas Day 1886. It is presented in velvety black-and-white tones that reminded me of the iconic Guinness adverts of the 1990s, with a dramatisation of the distillery's construction framed by lingering shots of the dirt-streaked, lined faces of the Grant family working "with their bare hands" and a voiceover in a warm Scottish burr that reiterates the tradition, integrity, and quality of the Glenfiddich brand as embodied by the honest toil and humble beginnings of its founding family. In all of its marketing, Glenfiddich is keen to get across that it owes its success not only to its specific ingredients, maturation process, and distillers' skill but most importantly to the fact that it is one of the few Scotch malts that is still a family business. This *is* notable, since many other major single malt brands are now owned by multinational companies including Diageo (Talisker, Lagavulin), Pernod Ricard (The Glenlivet, Chivas Regal), and LVMH Moët Henessey Louis Vuitton (Glenmorangie), though it does rather pass over the fact that William Grant & Sons make not only Glenfiddich but also the blended whisky Grant's, the single malt Balvenie, and a range of other products including the Irish whiskey Tullamore Dew, Reyka Icelandic vodka, and Hendrick's gin.

This spirit of inheritance and kinship is not confined to blood ties but extends to the workers in the distillery. For example, Glenfiddich's Malt Master—at the time of writing, the aptly named Brian Kinsman—is described thus on the company's website:

> Innate skill, drive and dedication underlie a Malt Master's ability to nose, taste and develop exceptional whiskies. Generations ago, our Malt Masters introduced marrying to smooth out fluctuations in flavour naturally occurring in maturing whiskies. Once whiskies have reached maturity, they are combined in oak marrying tuns. Here, spirits from different casks mellow and gather great consistency and harmony until our Malt Master decides they are ready for bottling. This knowledge has been passed down by Malt Masters through the ages—so you can enjoy over 125 years of wisdom in every glass.[4]

Although not all distilleries practice marrying—the combining of different runs of spirit in special casks to even out their subtly different flavours and so produce a consistent product—they do all routinely employ the romantic and generative rhetoric of distilling, from capturing the "heart" of the distillate to the use of "virgin casks," "pure" spring water, and, of course, the description of the spirit that naturally evaporates during maturation as "the angel's share."

What Glenfiddich readily demonstrates is the importance of place, tradition, kinship, and relationships between people and non-human organisms in the making of this luxury consumer good. And this is important, not only because whisky is such a vital contributor to the national economy but also because making whisky is also a way of making Scotland—or, at least, one version of Scotland.[5]

Origin Stories

Alternative living these days is more likely to refer
to the fact that you've bolted a solar panel to your
roof rather than undertaken any practical critique
of the nuclear family.

—*Nina Power*

The Lost Minke Whale

Early in August 2007, a minke whale calf was stranded in Fraserburgh harbour, fifty miles east of Spey Bay at the mouth of the Moray Firth. Minke whales, recognisable from their very small dorsal fins, are the most common type of whale to be spotted in the Moray Firth and are therefore thought of as the "local" whale species. Fraserburgh is a busy industrial fishing port whose harbour is usually crammed with enormous state-of-the-art deep-sea trawlers. This calf had swum unexpectedly into the harbour, following a trawler, and was stuck there for three days, apparently too disoriented to swim back out. In my discussions about the case with local people, many mentioned reports that an adult minke, which quickly became referred to as "the mother," had been spotted swimming in the sea outside the harbour wall during this time.

This unusual incident attracted both local and national attention, with people of all ages crowding around the harbour walls to see the whale. As Severin Carrell, *The Guardian*'s Scotland correspondent, put it, "Since the whale surfaced, Fraserburgh has discovered a new industry: eco-tourism. Car parks are busy with families unpacking cameras. Harbour authorities have erected crowd barriers and a sign stating: 'Whale watching: entry to piers at own risk.'"[1] Amongst these well-meaning onlookers, one young man took things too far, stripping to his underwear and jumping into the water to swim with the whale, emerging after thirty minutes to be arrested by the police.

Local conservation groups sprang into action to try and coax the calf back out to the open sea. They assumed that the calf was unable to get out of the harbour because it was disoriented and that human activities—exemplified by the heavy-duty fishing boats moored there—were interfering in its ability to use echolocation to escape. Amongst those involved in the rescue effort, there was a great deal of discussion about whether intervention was appropriate, with many worrying that their attempts to drive the whale out with underwater noise would be too distressing.[2] Eventually, just as the humans began to lose hope that they could rescue the whale, it followed a small flotilla of dinghies out to sea. Willow and one of the residential volunteers were in one of these boats and enjoyed the chance to experience a hands-on cetacean rescue. They returned to Spey Bay that evening to a hero's welcome.

In Spey Bay, there was plenty of discussion about the Fraserburgh minke calf. In contrast to the sperm whale stranding I described in the prologue, this was not only a chance to make a hands-on effort to help a whale in distress but a successful one that offered hope of salvation for the whale but also, symbolically, for the human community who had rescued it. This in fact echoes another difference between these two species of whale, as sperm whales are officially classified as "vulnerable" whilst minke whales are of "least concern" according to the International Union for Conservation of Nature's Red List of Threatened Species. In a context in which adults are thought of as having a responsibility to care for the environment that future generations will inherit, the fact that this case involved a stranded calf, rather than an adult, undoubtedly gave urgency to the rescue efforts, not only because it was seen as more vulnerable but because whales and dolphins need to re-produce successfully in order to escape endangerment, so any threat to a calf that has not had a chance to reproduce seems doubly tragic.

The distant figure of the calf's putative mother waiting in the nearby firth, apparently unable to help it back from its reckless path into the harbour, added a particular poignancy to this stranding story. People assumed that the calf would be all the more distressed because of its separation from its "mother" and that reuniting them would be the best, and perhaps only, way to ensure its survival. Indeed, once it finally swam back out into the firth they rapidly lost interest, based on their assumption that it had returned to the safety of its mother, pod, and home, and so no longer needed human assistance.

In identifying themselves with particular species, people draw upon and reformulate ideas about those specific animals' characteristics, which are, of course, no more "natural" than humans' ideas about themselves.[3] I often heard staff in the wild-life centre describing cetacean pods as if they were communities of extended nuclear families, especially when they were talking to children. In Spey Bay, dolphins and whales stand for particular ideas about nature, and humans' part in it, as well as modelling good interpersonal (or interspecies) relations. Popularly, and in Spey Bay, dolphins and whales are thought of as highly social, intelligent, and protective of their young, and these are qualities that people in Spey Bay also appreciate in humans.

The story of the lost minke calf and the protective behaviour towards calves amongst sperm whales that I described in the prologue both point to a particularly important kind of relation-ship of responsibility and care—that between mother and child. In interviews and conversations with people in Spey Bay, I did not explicitly ask them about maternal bonding,[4] but it came up again and again—especially in relation to two issues: surro-gacy and the differences between motherhood and fatherhood. In this chapter I will outline how people in Spey Bay and Moray thought about the relationship between maternal bonding and gender differences in parenting, before going on to discuss how one particular form of ART, surrogacy, troubles ideas about motherhood, maternal responsibility, and maternal bonding in the next chapter. I begin here by outlining two women's experiences of giving birth.

Birth Plans

Just twenty miles west along the coast from Spey Bay is a pretty village called Hopeman, where Erin, Duncan, and their daughter, Rosie, live in a one-storey cottage with a small patio garden. When I first visited northeast Scotland, a few months before starting fieldwork, I had viewed a flat just at the end of their road. As the owner showed me around, he made sure to point out that the first-floor kitchen window was a good vantage point for looking out to sea. "Sometimes, I've even seen dolphins while I'm doing the washing up," he told me.

Despite not succumbing to this tempting selling point, I found myself in Hopeman not long after arriving in northeast Scotland anyway. I had been on the telephone with my dad, who told me that an old friend of his, Duncan, and his family had recently moved there. He gave me their number and encouraged me to get in touch. I dialled the number he had given me shortly afterwards and Erin answered. She quickly invited me over to dinner the following week. That first dinner was the beginning of a series of invitations, and I went over during the day to spend time with Erin and Rosie, chatting over lunch or tea, or strolling down to the sea, many times. She had already taken Rosie to Spey Bay Wildlife Centre a few times by the time we met and greatly supported their cause, so she was pleased when I started volunteering there.

Erin is Duncan's second wife. He has adult children from his previous marriage; Erin was in her early thirties. They had expected that they would not have children of their own as Erin had had a car accident in her teens and her doctors told her then that, as a consequence of her abdominal injuries, she was unlikely to ever have children naturally. She told me that this had made her decide to focus on having a good career. Erin's parents died whilst she was young and she had given up a place to study at Cambridge University to look after her younger brothers. She later trained as a mental health nurse, during which time she met Duncan. Erin and Duncan had never considered pursuing ART to have a child together because they are practicing Catholics[5] and so, whilst they see themselves as liberal, modern Catholics who would not stop someone else from accessing medical treatments for infertility or from using contraception, they do not believe it is right for them. They looked into adoption quite seriously but had to abandon the idea after they were told by social workers that Duncan was too old to adopt.

Erin proudly told me that their wedding cost only £500, including the budget airline flights to Italy for their honeymoon, which is where she got pregnant. She greatly enjoyed her surprise pregnancy and described it as quite straightforward; the only negative points that she could recall were missing wine and mayonnaise. She did observe, however, that once her "bump" became very visible, her colleagues at work took her less seriously.

Rosie's birth was less straightforward. She was eventually born three weeks overdue, after several failed attempts to induce labour. By this point, she had become distressed and the medical team decided to perform an emergency caesarean section. Rosie spent the first three days of her life in a Special Care Baby Unit on oxygen therapy. Erin was, understandably, very distressed that her child was so unwell and her health was out of her hands, but she made a full recovery. Once Rosie was stabilised and they all went home, Erin found herself angry and disappointed that she had not been able to have the "natural," low-intervention birth she had planned. Telling me about it, she recalled how much emphasis had been put on designing a birth plan with the midwife earlier in her pregnancy and joked that the only use they had put it to in the end was "as toilet paper."

//

Some of the same tensions between knowledge, expectation, and control that Erin experienced characterised Jenny's birth story. She lives in a one-storey cottage near the sea with her partner, Paul, and their dog in Lossiemouth, which lies on the coast in between Hopeman and Spey Bay. Jenny is a senior social worker with decades of experience. She and Paul got together in later life; they both had families earlier on, and between them they have five adult children. Jenny's experience of giving birth to her twin sons was highly traumatic. Her pregnancy was "natural," in the sense that she and her husband at the time had no technological assistance to conceive, but because of failings in her care, she ended up having a great deal of intervention in the birth. Her story is best told in her own words, and it starts with her going into labour prematurely:

> Well, it was a great shock, because I was only six months pregnant. So the whole thing was an emergency, it was rushed, it was very scary because it was at that point that they discovered I was having twins and they couldn't hear the heartbeats, they thought that the two foetuses might be dead. And that was told to me, so the whole thing was extremely traumatic. I heard the phrase, "How many babies do you think you're having?" I'll always remember that. I felt like a rabbit lying there, thinking "oh my god" and I think, being a new mum, I had read all the books about what was supposed to happen during childbirth, gestation-wise, and had invested a bit in getting a bit further on in the pregnancy before thinking about viability. So I knew at that time I was at the very edges of what might be termed viable for one baby, let alone two. But I happened to give birth in the premier unit in the country—I was visiting somebody in Oxford and they had the best unit then in the whole country. But my two babies were actually put on lifesaving equipment there that meant that I witnessed a couple whose

baby was refused the chance of a life because my two babies were in the most specialised beds they'd got. So there were a whole catalogue of things that were happening that were very difficult.

When I was going through my pregnancy, I had a local GP where I was living then, in Birmingham, and she was lovely. I had a lot of problems around sickness because, unbeknownst to me, I was carrying twins and sickness is quite a reasonable indicator for a multiple birth, which I didn't know. I never had a scan. So I felt I had a good inter-personal relationship with my GP, but when I look back in retrospect, I wonder why, you know, the fact the I was carrying twins wasn't picked up. My husband at that time was a twin himself, so I think back now and I think that what happened in fact was, I was presenting with problems of sickness and I was given a drug called Debendox. You trust in your GP and I took Debendox because I was losing weight whilst pregnant rather than putting it on, and when my boys were born, one of them had a birth deformity, a huge mass on his arm, that was horrible, it looked really awful, it was gruesome to look at, and they couldn't operate on it. And it turned out that, it was disclosed to me over a period of time, that the drug Debendox was withdrawn in America and there were lawsuits in America where people successfully took the producers of the drug to court, and lit-igation.[6] That never happened in Britain, but I understand that it could've done. And I met several parents in those first few years with children with similar deformities and they'd all taken Debendox. So the treatment that I did have, whilst at the time I was happy with it, subsequently, looking back, I was quite dissatisfied with it.

. . . When my boys were born, I was actually caring for somebody who I loved a great deal who was dying, so the whole process of becoming a mother was not surrounded by the usual trappings of what one expects. It wasn't a de-light. I didn't know I was having twins, let alone one that was handicapped and [that they] were going to be in hospital with very profound needs for a very long time—the whole thing was not what I felt it should've been like. The "should haves," I had to throw out the window.

Fortunately, the experiences of Erin and Jenny, which happened two decades apart and in different parts of the UK, are not typical, and by recounting them here I do not intend to suggest that they are representative of women's birth experiences in Britain. They are interesting, though, in what they say about these women's ambivalence about medical and technological intervention in the birth process and, specifically, the importance of naturalness, knowledge, and care in their aspirations for a good birth. Sociologists and anthropologists have analysed the increasing medicalisation of birth in much of the Western world from the twentieth century onwards and feminist scholars have critiqued the masculine-biased medical establishment for wresting control over pregnancy and birth from pregnant and labouring women.[7] The increasing proliferation of information and advice about pregnancy, labour, and parenting can undermine women's sense of their own expertise and embodied knowledge and lead to a moralising view that women who resist medical advice, for example, by having a home birth for their first child or refusing medication during labour in pursuit of a "natural" birth, are "bad" mothers who would put their own desires above the well-being of their child.[8] The literature on the medicalisation of pregnancy and birth also reminds us that there was already a considerable amount of technological and medical "intervention" in reproduction before the advent of ART.

Both Jenny and Erin shared a sense that their expectations about what their children's births would be like were lost in their doctors' understandable yet limited focus on their medical treatment. Whilst Jenny had to throw her ideas about what her sons' birth should have been like "out the window," Erin's birth plan seemed to be no better than "toilet paper" once she entered the labour ward. In both their cases, their babies were in severe danger and both Jenny and Erin recognise that their children probably would not have survived without the medical attention they got, yet in telling their birth stories, they also made it clear that they felt there had been failings in their care along the way.

For Jenny in particular, the fact that she did not know she was carrying twins until she was in premature labour epitomises the lack of information, or misinformation, she felt she was subject to during her pregnancy. On the one hand, she described a good interpersonal relationship with her GP and attributed the standard of care in the hospital in which she gave birth to saving the lives of her sons. But on the other hand, she implied that the GP failed her by missing the clues that she was having twins and prescribing a drug that Jenny felt was harmful. From Jenny's point of view, her embodied experience, her husband's genetic makeup, and the testimony of other people who had taken Debendox were all overridden by her GP's authority and expertise as a medical practitioner.

In the previous chapter, I described the concerns of people in Spey Bay that overreliance on technology to conceive children might lead to increasing infertility and even species endangerment. Jenny told me, quite casually, that both the fact that she gave birth by caesarean and that it was in the hospital made her experience of giving birth "unnatural." The ideas and ideals Jenny and Erin had about giving birth demonstrate the dilemmas of managing a "natural' process. Their experiences of giving birth in very difficult circumstances show the tricky tension between the desire to let nature take its course and assisting nature when it fails, which can lead to a loss of control and a sense of distance from what is natural. These dilemmas are undoubtedly heightened by the fact that they live in a milieu in which parenting, and scrutiny of parenting, is intensified and in which parents—and mothers in particular—are thought to bear ultimate responsibility for their children's welfare and development.[9]

Responsibility

As a local volunteer at the wildlife centre, I helped out at a number of events, including, on one occasion, dressing in a dolphin costume and walking around a local boat festival with a collection tin whilst my colleagues staffed a stall with activities for children and information about whales and dolphins. I was surprised and rather touched by how many young children, mostly girls, rushed up to me in my dolphin outfit, eager to put their pocket money into my tin. I was struck by how concerned about the state and future of the environment they and their parents and others I chatted with that day were. There was similar concern amongst people I met whilst helping out at another event a few months later, this time in Aberdeen. There, I helped supervise children making posters about threats to cetaceans and their habitats, which many of them took to enthusiastically. But when I explained what the children were doing to a group of passing visitors, one mother with a child of about six years old wrinkled her nose and said, gesturing to her daughter, "I'm not sure I want her to know about things like that, I don't want to fill her innocent ears with things like that." For Jenny, Erin, and the people who work in the wildlife centre, having children is not only a natural process but also one that activates a unique ethic of responsibility. Most basically, as the Aberdonian woman's concerns about exposing her daughter to talk of endangerment suggests, this is the responsibility to keep children safe. The everyday care of children could, then, perhaps be framed as the short-term counterpart of their long-term responsibility to protect future generations.

For both Jenny and Erin, their children's births were also a rebirth for them. Jenny said, "I had absolutely no idea of the profundity of what it would mean in my life," whilst Erin described motherhood as being "hit" with a "massive notion of responsibility, which just explodes when the child arrives" and as "an immense emotional relationship that is tied in with a huge amount of responsibility." When I interviewed Erin and asked about her experience of being a mother, she described some of the practical ways in which motherhood had transformed her life. She said, "It changes your goals and ambitions . . . it alters your perception on your life and where it's going," and in my many interactions with them, I observed how important Rosie was in her everyday decisions. Erin had given up work to look after Rosie but was studying for a degree with the Open University. She told me that although her course was important to her, if she had to weigh up perfecting an essay against spending time with Rosie, Rosie would always be her priority.

Both Erin and Jenny described motherhood as a balance of rewards and sacrifices, based on the unique sense of responsibility that characterises being a parent. Jenny's partner, Paul, also described being a parent as a "two-edged sword." He said, "It means happiness and fulfilment, but it's also responsibility and worry. Even though my eldest is thirty-two and my youngest is twenty, they're always your children and even though they're grown up, they still might have problems that you feel you need to take part in in some way." I asked Paul if he felt becoming a father had changed his identity and he said, "Getting married was like one step on the maturity ladder, [but] actually having a child—it's like a reality check and I knew I needed to take some responsibility for the life and chop my hair off and get a job, get a house, and all that. It changed me a lot."

Richard is a father of two and stepfather to three. Like Paul, when I asked about his experience of fatherhood, he said, "It made me grow up." He continued, "Children or babies make adults of their parents, you know, suddenly you're faced with the reality of being responsible for this little bundle of human life, and you have to grow up really fast." He did admit, though, that this sense of responsibility was different with his stepchildren: "I think the real cop-out with stepchildren is that you can, you can finally say, 'Well, that's not my responsibility, this is not my child,' if you want to get away with something, which I sometimes did! I think it's different."

All four of these parents described parenthood, and the responsibility that came with it, as changing them, and as we saw in the first chapter, people in Spey Bay who did not have children also anticipated the profound way in which parenthood would affect their lives if and when the time came. The younger women who worked and volunteered in the wildlife centre seemed to be particularly acutely aware of this, which reflects their shared assumption that they, rather than their partners, would be their children's primary caregivers. People were explicit and reflexive about the fact that the responsibility of parenthood brings about a new personal ethic, which is seen as having costs and rewards. As Erin put it,

> You feel very proud, you know, [to have] somebody that's related to you, that you love, that you've created, so immensely proud and it's immensely positive because you are given a chance for another identity if you like. You're given a chance to be somebody's mummy, or somebody's parent. So that is sort of a time where I sort of felt—I'm sure some of it was hormonal—euphoric, at the idea that you can re-create yourself.
>   . . . I'd lie if I didn't say that there are sacrifices, there are compromises that come with being a parent and they sometimes can be really, really difficult and costly. They can be costly. I mean, you know, it's not life and death, but sometimes you feel that, whether it's the old you that you don't recognise so much anymore, you know, as you change and as you evolve and become a parent, there are times when you sort of get glimpses of, "if I wasn't a parent, I might be doing this" or "I might take this opportunity or that opportunity."

Implicit in both Jenny's and Erin's descriptions of their birth experiences was a sense that the trust they had put in their doctors had been misplaced and that the responsibility for their, and their children's, care had not been taken seriously enough. In the previous chapter, I described people's shared aspiration that children will grow up in a stable environment and suggested that this was related to their wider ethical values of caring for other people and their environment. The unique responsibility of parenthood is one that comes from making quotidian life-and-death decisions on behalf of another, dependent person. The frustration that Erin and Jenny both felt over the way in which information and control were withheld from them during the births of their children was a hard lesson in this.

Parenthood brings a unique sense of responsibility, which both mothers and fathers feel. However, there is a vital difference in how people perceived motherhood as compared to fatherhood, which is the assumption that the physical and embodied experience of pregnancy and birth will lead to a special, unique bond between a mother and child. Though on the one hand this sense of a special relationship between mother and child valorises motherhood, it can also reproduce the ideology that mothers have a greater sense of responsibility for their children and consequently make the most naturally predisposed, and therefore best, parents.

A Vital Difference

The story of the lost minke whale calf in Fraserburgh harbour illustrates the point that, as people in Spey Bay see it, compromising natural phenomena like the bond between a whale and her calf causes pain and suffering and threatens death. The assumption that the lost minke whale calf would be saved by simply being reunited with its "mother" points to an aspect of parenthood that is as important for humans as for cetaceans: the maternal bond. Here I will outline people's experiences and observations about this phenomenon and specifically its relationship to bodily experience.

The purchase that the mother-child relationship has had on psychological theory suggests its deep significance to how we conceptualise identity, sexuality, kinship, gender, health, and well-being. From Freud to Bowlby, psychoanalysts and psychologists have assumed that unhealthy attachments between mother and child create higher risks of mental, and even physical, ill health for the child later in life. Attachment theory may have lost some of its former authority for psychologists, but ideas about mother-child bonding are inherent in popular parenting culture,[10] and current social and public policy is informed by an assumption that a positive early experience of parent-child (but usually mother-child) bonding is vital to giving children the right start in life.[11]

Whether or not they had children, people in Spey Bay described the maternal bond as a psychological and emotional attachment that arises naturally and inevitably out of the embodied experience of pregnancy. They all thought of the maternal bond as compelling mothers towards particular kinds of behaviours and relationships, including specifically the ethic of responsibility I outlined earlier. As she told me in an interview whilst Rosie was at nursery school, Erin started feeling a bond forming with her daughter from the moment she had a positive pregnancy test:

> For me, part of this special bond was, all the way through the pregnancy, my intestines were being kicked to bits, I was the one on the loo twenty times a day, but it was actually something that Duncan could only participate in to a point. You know, I could say, "Ooh look, come and feel this baby kicking," but you already have a psychological and emotional bond . . . if you like, I got a nine-month head start on the bloke concerned and I think you can't compete with that and I think that makes mummies that carry their own children special in their own right.

By emphasising her intimate, physical connection to her daughter through her phrase "a nine-month head start," Erin located her bond with her in both a different time and place, which her husband, Duncan, could not access because of his different physiological relationship to her.

People made repeated references to the nine-month period of pregnancy when I talked to them about motherhood, and it was generally accepted that the uniqueness of this physical experience would create a similarly unique bond. Charlotte, for example, said, "There's nothing else in the world like it, is there? Nobody else can do what we can, potentially. . . . I can't imagine what that sort of bond must feel like, when you carry someone for nine months and then, you know, give birth to them. I just can't, it's completely unique."

Nina comes from the Highlands and her partner is in the RAF. She told me in an interview that she planned to have children in the future and that if she had trouble conceiving "naturally" she would prefer to use assisted conception to adopting because she was concerned that it would not be "enough" for her:

> Yeah, it's just carrying on the family line, I guess, and I don't know if you'd ever have quite the same bond with a child that you'd adopted, even from a baby, with a child that had actually come from you and you'd had inside you for nine months. I think that's—it might be different for men and women—because, you know carrying a child for nine months, you're bonding with it for all that time. Whereas, adoption, you don't really get the whole thing, you just get the baby, you don't get the whole experience that goes with it. I think just being pregnant, before you even get the child, is a big part of it, and something that every woman maybe wants to experience.

For Nina, being pregnant is an important part of being a woman, but carrying and giving birth to a child are also about safeguarding the formation of a bond between mother and child.

In her research amongst mothers of different ages in Scotland, Kelly Davis found that bonding with their children was something that mothers expected to happen but that entailed work and time.[12] For the mothers she interviewed "maternal instinct" was on the one hand a complex of emotions, especially protectiveness and deep love, which seemed to arise naturally, whilst on the other hand it was the intimate and personal knowledge of one's child that comes through knowing and caring for her. Based on their own observations and experiences, people in Spey Bay similarly suggested that bonds between mothers and children need to be worked on, implying that although maternal bonding may be something that begins "naturally," its full development is not always inevitable or automatic but must be nurtured.

People were evenly split about whether they thought that a mother's bond to a child would be stronger or more special than a father's throughout their child's life or if this difference would eventually even out. Though people disagreed about how far-reaching the effects of the mother-child bond might be in time, they generally assumed that the physical, hormonal, and emotional realities of pregnancy and labour offer the right conditions for a "special" relationship to grow between mother and child. Some people thought that the maternal bond caused mothers and fathers to play different roles as parents. Amy told me the following:

> I think the mum has a stronger bond at the beginning, but I think that's just to do with carrying the baby around for nine months. But then, the dad seems to be kind of more doting and spoils the child a lot more sometimes. So, I think the mother—it's kind of stereotypical—but the mother always seems to be the more kind of practical one and does the basic care of the child, whereas the dad is usually the one that comes in and spoils the children and plays with them.

Amy was clearly aware that these differences she had observed in how women and men approach parenting were "stereotypical," and many of her friends and colleagues were keen to point out that they thought that men and women could be jointly involved in parenting and they had observed that amongst their peers who had children, the fathers tended to be much more "hands on" than were fathers in their parents' generation. Lauren, who talked about the "natural limits" of female fertility in the last chapter and is a good friend of Amy's, thought that typically there would be differences in the ways in which men and women parent "because women can actually carry the children," and she thought that women tend towards "natural, responsive nurturing" because of their capacity to breastfeed. Lauren observed that her male friends often expressed a desire to have "a larger role" in the lives of their children but that generally speaking it was mothers who tended to stay at home with the children. Her partner, Jack, agreed with her that people of their generation were likely to aim for more equal roles in parenting. He did think, however, that "women have a sort of innate desire to have kids more than a lot of men do."

There is a subtle but important difference between believing that fathers can be "more involved" or can contribute "more equally" to parenting and believing that there is no reason why women or men should be thought of as the primary caregivers of children by virtue of their gender. What seems to be vital in this is the "nine-month head start" that Erin described, the sense that gestating another person will naturally lead to the formation of a special bond that is the basis for a lasting and unique relationship of care and responsibility.

When I asked Jenny to reflect on whether women and men approach parenthood differently, she said that she thought these roles were "different but hopefully complementary." Jenny's experience of giving birth was one in which her expectations of what the experience would be like were upturned, and this was exacerbated by the fact that when they were born, both of her sons needed a great deal of medical support to survive, plus one of them had a physical deformity and, they later discovered, learning difficulties. In discussing parenting roles more generally, she pinpointed a "breakdown" between expectation and reality as a source of difficulty for many other parents, too.

Jenny described parenting as more "complicated" now, because people's expectations of what it takes to be ideal parents are too far removed from "reality," and in making this claim she pointed to her own expertise as a senior social worker:

> *Jenny:* I think how very difficult it is for people who have all these pre-birth conceptions of what the idealised version of being a parent might be, and whether they're a drug addict or whether they're a middle-class citizen, people are gonna have expectations, hopes for that child, and dreams. Then the reality of, like, perhaps sleepless nights, and a change in their couple relationship if it's their first time—'cause I think that's crucial—and the stresses on relationships generally that exist in society now, they all impact on that parenting role. . . . It's just so complicated now. It was probably a lot easier back, in some regards, back when there were defined gender roles.

> *KD:* Do you think so?

> *Jenny:* I do, yeah. I'm not saying that I think there were necessarily all good things about that, because I can see why society's evolved to the point we have—[*laughs*] "evolved" [is a] questionable word—but there's a huge breakdown in, a gap, I think, between expectation and what is reality for a lot of people. . . . I've dealt with a lot of families in my job, so I *know*, I understand in a very real way, how that's manifest[ed] itself. (Original emphasis)

During this interview, I was somewhat surprised to hear Jenny suggest that the "defined gender roles" of previous generations had made parenting easier, as it seemed like an uncharacteristically conservative view based on what I knew about her political and social attitudes more generally. I think she was not so much intending to criticise the idea of gender equality in itself but suggesting that new ideals can create new problems as people renegotiate entrenched social roles and divisions of labour.

This example also points to the different registers of interview data and ethnographic observations. By asking Jenny if she perceived gender differences in parenting during my interview with her, I was probably—if not entirely intentionally—inviting her to make a stronger claim than she might have, were we talking about a specific example. But it is also important to listen to Jenny's point here, which as she said was based in her considerable professional experience. Just as there is a gap between what people might say in a formal interview and what they would say in an informal conversation (or in different conversations at different times), there is a gap between "expectations" and "reality" or, to put it another way, norms and practices in people's lives. Rather than necessarily stating a political position, Jenny was here reflecting on her experience and empathising with the difficulties that many people face in reconciling what is expected of them as good partners, parents, kin, or citizens and what they can manage in reality.

Conclusion

Erin described motherhood as a creative process. Her pride in creating a child was evident in her description of what it meant to her to have become a mother, but clearly it was not just a child that she created but a new sense of herself—and perhaps even a new self. Key to this is the new ethic of responsibility, the reorienting of her life towards the protection and nurturance of another human being whom she has created. She described having a "nine-month head start" on bonding with her daughter compared to her husband because of the ways in which pregnancy took over her physical experience. In discussing maternal bonding, people were rarely specific about which particular aspects of biological motherhood led to the formation of a maternal bond. Many mentioned pregnancy (which is of course a diverse experience with a huge range of physical effects) and giving birth, but some also mentioned breastfeeding or the experience of emotional reactions to crying babies. In a sense, though, this is the point—that becoming a parent is an experience that affects every aspect of life and the physical characteristics of this are perhaps only the most obvious. In previous chapters I noted that people rarely talked of genetic inheritance in expressing their concerns about ART or the future of kinship. Here, in people's ideas about maternal bonding, which might seem like an obvious place to hear about inheritance, people talked about making or creating a child, and they framed this in terms of biophysical experience, yet they did not use the language of genetics or shared substance to express this. Perhaps this is because it is too obvious to be worth mentioning—or perhaps because the physical experience of natural processes has sufficient explanatory power.

In describing their experiences and observations of parenthood, people in Spey Bay focused on biophysical experience and the novelty of having responsibility for a dependent person in determining and characterising this phenomenon. The link between these two is the bond between parent and child, which they expected to be strongest for mothers, based on the different extent to which parenthood affects them at the bodily level. Whilst they were generally supportive of gender equality, in talking about the maternal bond, people in Spey Bay made a claim for the specialness of motherhood based on gendered biological difference. They saw this specialness as bringing rewards and costs. By associating the responsibilities of parenthood with the maternal bond, which is seen as being activated by the physical intimacy of pregnancy and birth, it becomes both a biological and ethical expectation for a mother to form a close bond with her child and to therefore feel responsible for her care. This implies that the physical experience of pregnancy and labour will guide and motivate nurturance. It also has the effect of implying that women, because of their biology, are naturally equipped for parenthood. People did not dispute the idea that fathers should be "involved" in parenting and many thought that, over time, fathers could come to feel as close to their children as mothers, but the power of the idea that women *naturally* make good parents should not be underestimated, not least when it is held by people who are explicitly interested in protecting nature.

In the previous chapter, I discussed the critique some scholars have made of the discourse surrounding endocrine disrupting chemicals, highlighting how key players in the environmental movement have played on cultural anxieties about changing norms of gender and sexuality to bolster their case for protecting the environment from the "feminising" pollutants Jenny and others mentioned. Given the long association of the environmental movement with feminism and progressive politics, I suspect the heteronormativity of these campaigns is usually an unintended—if effective—consequence. Nonetheless, what this example and the example of maternal bonding discussed in this chapter both show is that, in seeking to protect "nature" and "natural" reproduction, people can end up protecting and reproducing established norms of gender and sexuality. This is because gender, sexuality, reproduction, and kinship have long been intimately associated with nature and biology.[13] In British culture, reproduction is thought of as the "facts of life," a natural process driven by evolutionary forces and shaped by biology.[14] Anything that seems to denature "normal" gender or sexuality, like pollutants that cause species to change sex, therefore seems like a threat to nature itself.

In discussing Jenny's and Erin's birth stories earlier in this chapter, I noted the tension they experienced between letting nature take its course and assisting nature when it failed. This echoes the ethical tension that people felt between sympathising with infertile people's desire to have children and their concern about the unintended consequences of excessive interference in natural processes and Sophie's dilemma between her "right-on politics" and sense of what was natural in relation to the prospect of postmenopausal women using IVF to conceive, as well as the practical discussions about how far to intervene in saving the minke whale calf in Fraserburgh harbour. As the idea of the stable environment suggests, part of making a good life is finding the right balance between competing values and motivations. In this chapter, I have shown the important part that ideas of nature, biology, and embodied experience play in forming people's perceptions of parenting and particularly motherhood, which is exemplified by the maternal bond. In the next chapter, I will explore what happens when the naturalness of the maternal bond is challenged.

// *Arrivals*

The first time I spotted a cetacean in Scotland, I was in Macduff in Aberdeenshire. I rented a flat there when I arrived for fieldwork. Chris and I were out walking around the small fishing town. Walking was one of our main activities then, when we arrived in Scotland and before I had started volunteering in Spey Bay. When it was really cold, we would drink hot chocolate with a nip of whisky in it when we got back home.

That day wasn't in fact the first time I had seen a cetacean in the wild, though my first sighting had only been a month or so earlier. Chris and I had been on holiday to Mexico and on our last day there we had rented kayaks and gone out into the Pacific. The dolphins came so close I started to worry about them capsizing us. The proximity made me realise their size and might.

Back in Macduff, it was an overcast day, one where the clouds are so darkly grey and indistinguishable from each other that when you look out of the window first thing in the morning, you know there is no hope of direct sunshine all day; you can only console yourself that at least it might not rain. There are a lot of days like that in northeast Scotland, days when you fantasise about a wing chair and an open fire, though there are also many days when the wind blows so hard the clouds have no choice but to evaporate and reveal the sun after all. Sometimes it is simply sunny, warm, and not too windy. There were lots of days like that later that summer, which suffered—or, in the case of Scotland, enjoyed—a Europe-wide heatwave.

That particular grey day, we were walking on the brow of the hill on which the town sits, making our way down towards the park by the Knowes Hotel, when we looked up and out to sea. Right in our line of vision, there was something, a small dark shape against the brown-grey water of the Moray Firth. Chris identified it as a minke whale. I had wondered, before, whether I would definitely recognise what I was seeing when I finally did see a cetacean in the Moray Firth. It was only once I had seen that small black fin, so unmistakeable, that I realised that that was an unnecessary concern. I was exhilarated. I began to see for myself what the fuss was about, how some people can end up devoting their lives to saving cetaceans. Something about seeing one in the wild, yet so close to where people were going about their ordinary lives, was so strange as to seem magical.

//

I made several first trips to Spey Bay. The time that I really arrived was in fact my fourth time there. After living in Macduff for a few months and struggling to make connections with people there, I decided that voluntary work might be a good way to meet local people. I had visited Spey Bay and the wildlife centre on my first visit to the area, a recce before starting fieldwork, when I went to have a look at the area and find a place to live. Chris and I had walked along the Spey and the beach there a few times since. Whilst I was investigating what opportunities there might be to volunteer in the area, it came back to me. I sent an email asking whether they were looking for volunteers. An enthusiastic response arrived in my inbox, asking me to pop in for a chat. I drove over to the wildlife centre a few days later. It was another grey day and the place looked deserted, but as I approached from the car park, I was greeted by Sophie, who took me on a tour of the centre and the office, where we met Andrew, who had just started working as a residential volunteer.

Sophie, Andrew, and I went to Sophie's house, where Sophie made tea and got a packet of biscuits out. She told me about the work of the wildlife centre and about the different roles of the residential volunteers and the local volunteers; the latter is what I would be. I always found it amusing to be referred to as a local volunteer, though by the time I was myself living in Sophie's house, it didn't jar quite so much. By then I felt part of the place, or at least that the place was a part of me. Sophie asked me about my research and seemed quite intrigued. We chatted a little about life in Spey Bay and I was struck by Sophie's warmth and enthusiasm. Both she and Andrew made me feel welcome and useful. For the first time since arriving in northeast Scotland, I started to feel like something was happening, like my fieldwork was really beginning.

As well as being British and having my own kinship links to Scotland, I was at home in Spey Bay in the sense that I have a great deal of sympathy for the environmental movement. Living amongst people who are explicitly concerned about climate change and marine conservation has left its own effects on me. Although people never quite completely forgot that I was a Londoner and an academic, I did fit in politically and ethically in Spey Bay (and indeed, amongst my academic and Londoner friends, I am sometimes teased for being a bit "granola"). I proved my place in this community of like-minded people by showing my willingness to muck in and to give things a go, such as agreeing to don an ill-fitting dolphin costume and rattle a fund-raising tin at a boat festival in support of the overarching cause of cetacean conservation and environmentalism. Of course these were not entirely altruistic acts of mine, since they were also done in the cause of my fieldwork.

Kay Milton points out that one problem for social scientists who engage with environmentalism is that it is an evolving cause in which we are, as people and as advocates for other people, inevitably implicated.[1] With the mainstreaming of environmentalist ethics, every choice we make in the supermarket, and indeed the decision to set foot in a supermarket in the first place, is a political and ethical one, whether in our personal lives or during fieldwork. Environmentalism raises the question of how we study something we are part of, though this is hardly a new one for ethnographers, especially those of us working in our "own" cultures. I wonder if one reason why more social scientists have not engaged with environmentalism as an object of study is not only its global nature but that many of us feel a great deal of political and ethical sympathy with the cause. If this is so, it may also be a recognition of the fact that putting things into context has the "displacement effect"[2] of making them explicit and thereby exposing them to further analytic scrutiny and making them appear "only" cultural.

What is a good life for me? After a childhood spent in pleasant, quiet East Anglian villages, I moved to London at the first opportunity. I have spent most of my adult life in London. I love London—its vitality, its throttled pulse, its diversity, the way it feels like a slumbering dragon. Still, I came to feel at home in Spey Bay, which made me question just what my version of the good life is and whether it necessarily has to be located in a particular place at all. Of course I always knew I was there temporarily and that I would always, however close I became with the many friends I made in Spey Bay, be distanced by the fact that I was studying them.

In "The Ethics of Participant Observation," Nigel Rapport reflects on his experience in Wanet, Cumbria, and argues that ethnographic research should both "convey a sense of its own locatedness" and "express a sense of the emergence of its data through particular personal relations and particular discourses."[3] As he points out, there are no static, bounded, absolute objects of ethnographic analysis; no one follows one particular set of cultural or ethical rules in deciding how to live their life. Ethnography, then, creates new realities just as it creates new relations, and in so doing, Rapport suggests, it can take up an ethical position by juxtaposing the usual way in which a particular social world is described (or how it describes itself) against the description of the ethnographer.[4]

Because I did my fieldwork in the same country in which I was born and bred, I could be described as having done ethnography "at home," despite the fact that I had never set foot in Moray before 2005. For me, the fact that I did fieldwork somewhere where I felt at home—which, to be honest, was a complete surprise, as I had expected fieldwork to be hard, lonely, and even a little miserable—is more significant. It was not overfamiliarity with the language or prevailing social norms that I had to overcome in mastering a comfortable distance from the

people I studied but a strong sympathy with their everyday ethics. In this, my experience was very different from Rapport's,
who found that he had to conceal many of his true opinions
and important parts of his identity. Still, in coming to think
through the implications of everything that people said to me
during fieldwork, I have also had to accept where our ethics, and
politics, diverge.

Ties That Bind

> ... with unrelaxed and breathless eagerness
> I pursued nature to her hiding-places.
>
> —*Mary Shelley*

"As Nature Intended"?

In November 2006, I attended a hearing at the Highland Council regarding the proposed development of Whiteness Head, the site of a disused oil rig fabrication plant outside Inverness, into a residential and leisure site. On the day, I had had a desperate telephone call from Sophie asking if I could give her a lift to the meeting in Inverness. She had been called upon to represent the charity's objections to the development at the last minute since no one was available to travel up from their English headquarters. The charity was concerned about the effects of increased boat traffic on the cetacean population due to the large new marina that was planned as part of the development. Whiteness Head is very close to Chanonry Point, a spit of uninhabited land on the northern side of the Inner Moray Firth that is known in wildlife-watching circles along with Spey Bay as one of the most reliable places to spot the Moray Firth dolphins, with almost daily sightings at the height of summer.

Having driven Sophie to the council offices, I went in with her to lend moral support and had an opportunity to witness local political process firsthand. The council chambers are set up much like the Scottish Parliament, with councillors and interested parties seated in a hemicycle oriented towards the chairperson's desk. Their desks are equipped with power points for laptop computers and microphones that light up when in use. A further layer of public seating, without desks, encircles this. The councillors themselves were all white, male, and middle-aged and wore either dark business suits or more brightly coloured tweed suits. Apart from Sophie and me, the only women present were the chairperson's assistant and the representative from the Ministry of Defence (MoD). Sophie, the MoD representative, and I were also the only ones under thirty years old. Applicants and objectors were each allotted time slots of ten minutes, in accordance with the official guidelines for such hearings.[1] First to present was the representative for the applicants, who went to some pains to detail the amount of time, effort, and money the company had spent on every aspect of the plans as well the involvement of the architect, whom he consistently referred to as "Sir Terry" in a manner that suggested both deference and familiarity. Throughout, he emphasised "best practice" and the environmental and social credentials of the project.

After the developers spoke, the councillors were allowed to ask questions and seek clarifications about the proposal. The objectors then had their turn to speak. First was Jeff, a member of a local grassroots conservation group. He talked about his observations of dolphin behaviour and boat-based human-dolphin interaction, claiming authority through the amount of time he had spent observing cetaceans, to argue that further boat traffic would be detrimental to them. Sophie spoke next from a prepared statement, which gave clear reasons for the charity's objections and argued that developments such as this should not be treated in isolation when deciding on their likely ecological and environmental impact. Last to speak was the MoD representative, who spoke about the potential effect of the development on the operation of a nearby firing range.

The councillors were given a chance to ask questions and seek clarifications from the objectors next. Almost all of the questions were directed at Jeff and Sophie and centred on requesting statistical information, which Sophie had already noted was difficult to collect.[2] The councillors seemed unconvinced that increased boat traffic would be detrimental to the cetacean population, though this was largely based on general feeling rather than evidence, in contrast to their demands for "proof," as they put it, from the objectors to support their views. The chairperson remarked that he had observed no problems in the cetacean population on his most recent fishing trip in the Moray Firth, whilst another councillor said that he was old enough to remember when people had gone out fishing for herring on the firth and that that traffic seemed to have had no effect on the cetacean population. He concluded, "I'm concerned that we are suggesting that these dolphins and porpoises aren't as resilient as nature intended."

Next, the applicants were allowed to respond to the objections. They handed over to their "expert," a biologist from St. Andrews University. He asserted from the start that everything he said would be based on "scientific research and evidence," though he did not present any statistical evidence of the sort asked of the objectors, instead referring repeatedly to two papers he had written on the matter, which were not detailed in the proceedings of the hearing and which, it may not be far-fetched to assume, had not been read by most of the people present. When he had finished, the planning officer announced that the development had been approved to go forward for ministerial approval, subject to certain conditions. The hearing ended with a final session of questions from the councillors.

As people filtered out of the chamber, Sophie was approached by journalists from the local paper *The Press and Journal* (P&J) and the BBC. The chairman also came over to thank her for attending. Turning to me, he asked her, "Is this your wee assistant?"[3] He then asked the P&J journalist if he would rather talk to Sophie or him first, jovially pointing out that Sophie was clearly the more attractive choice. Sophie was unimpressed, and as I drove us back to Spey Bay she railed against the setup of the hearing, saying, "I don't want it to be like this, but I can't help but wonder if it would have made any difference to our case if I'd been a middle-aged man in a suit."

About six months later, Sophie and I were talking about a television programme that a few of our friends in Spey Bay had watched that set out to "debunk" climate change. We were both surprised that Amy had said that watching the programme had made her unsure about the effects of climate change. To me, Sophie observed that it can sometimes take very little for someone to change their mind and she suggested that as long as someone is presented as a scientist, his or her opinions will probably be accepted as credible. Sophie was frustrated that she had not seen the programme herself, telling me that if she had, she would have been able to take each point it made and argue against it. She said it reminded her of our experience at the Highland Council the previous December, remarking, "As long as you've got a scientist to support you, you can expect people to trust what you're saying."

Most of the wildlife centre's paid staff, including Sophie, in fact have a background in the biological sciences and they are involved in a range of scientific research, most of which focuses on collecting records of the numbers of cetaceans in the area through surveys, sightings data, and "Photo ID," where they take photographs of the dorsal fins of any dolphins sighted whilst guiding on wildlife-watching boats in order to identify them and record their movements. But in the Whiteness Head case, there was no opportunity to assert this and it seemed at the time that even if Sophie had peppered her account with statistical projections about the impact of the development on the welfare of the Moray Firth dolphins, her claims would have been found wanting, as the whole hearing seemed to be heading towards a foregone conclusion.

The councillors' comments about the natural resilience of cetaceans struck me forcefully at the time—not only because of their audacity and the fact that my ethnographic antennae tend to respond to any such overt characterisations of nature but also because of the authority over the natural world that they implied. Ostensibly the hearing was about whether or not to allow the economic and physical development of a particular site of land that fell within the Highland Council's jurisdiction. But it can be seen through another lens: that of what is at stake in making claims on and with nature, which is the main theme of this chapter. The meeting was like a card game in which the players were competing to have their view of nature accepted. Although I of course have my own biases, it seemed to me as I observed the meeting that some of the players' decks were stacked, not necessarily because of any nefarious intent but because of the ways in which claims about nature and the natural world are made to fit particular agendas and interests.

//

In the previous chapter, I showed how people in Spey Bay think of the maternal bond as a natural phenomenon that arises out of embodied experience. This once again suggests the salience of nature and biology in how people think and make claims about reproduction. However, in this chapter I will muddy the waters by training my focus onto their ideas about surrogacy. What happens to ideas of maternal bonding when a woman who has gestated and given birth to a child agrees to give her up to another person's care at birth? And what if she is also genetically related to that child?

One of the practical problems that surrogacy presents is the risk that the surrogate mother might decide to keep the baby. This is also an ethical question of whether or not surrogate mothers should form a bond with the children they carry for intended parents. When I discussed surrogacy with people in Spey Bay, this question emerged as the most problematic in their views about this practice. In this chapter, I will trace some of the connections and disconnections that emerged between how people thought about maternal bonding in terms of their own experience of non-technologically assisted reproduction, which I outlined in the previous chapter, and their thoughts about surrogacy. By taking this comparative approach, my aim is to contextualise their judgements of surrogacy and to show the contingent and strategic ways in which they drew upon the maternal bond.

The continued coverage of surrogacy arrangements in the media and the ongoing debate over surrogacy amongst feminists[4] show how this practice provokes intense social, ethical, and political anxieties.[5] This continues to this day, though the focus of research most recently has turned to the burgeoning transnational surrogacy industry. There is empirical evidence that surrogacy can be distressing and exploitative for those involved, and it has quite rightly received attention from bioethicists, from feminist scholars, and from the point of view of reproductive justice.[6] But for those not personally involved in surrogacy, like people in Spey Bay, the reason why it is so contentious is because it upturns taken-for-granted beliefs about the nature of motherhood and challenges normative ideas about kinship and femininity. Where once maternity seemed certain because a child's mother could only be the woman who had given birth to her, with surrogacy and egg donation, opportunities to have more than one "biological" mother seem to be opened up.[7] However, as Sarah Franklin has shown, despite the challenges that ART including surrogacy present to deeply held views about kinship, parenthood, and gender, in practice they often have the effect of reinforcing heteronormative models of family formation and conjugal relationships.[8]

In a time of ART, public concern about parenting, and more general fears about the future of the natural world and species endangerment, motherhood has become a focus for a range of wider anxieties about demographic change, shifting gender roles, and the well-being of future generations. In the next section I will analyse how people in Spey Bay drew on the maternal bond to make nuanced claims about motherhood and the ethics of surrogacy to show how "natural" concepts like the maternal bond are used contingently and strategically in ethical judgements about reproduction and parenting. Later in the chapter, I will remain with the example of surrogacy in order to explore the salience of altruism as a site of ethical value.

Scrambled Eggs

Although there are suggestions that informal surrogacy arrangements have taken place since ancient times, surrogacy decisively
entered the British public arena in the 1980s with the case of Kim
Cotton, the UK's first, and so far only, "commercial' surrogate
mother. Cotton, a married mother of two, carried a baby on behalf of a Swedish couple who paid her £6,500 in an arrangement
organised by an American surrogacy agency working in south-
east England, though in fact she received far more money for
selling her story to a newspaper (for which she was also vilified,
unlike the parents of Louise Brown, who similarly had an exclusive deal with the *Daily Mail*).[9] Fenella Cannell has argued that
Cotton was a culturally problematic figure because she had failed
to bond with the child she carried as a surrogate.[10] Despite the
fact that she was thereby fulfilling the obligation she had made to
the intended parents and the people who set up the arrangement,
in the contemporary uproar, her actions came to represent quintessentially "bad" and "unnatural" maternal behaviour.

With surrogacy, the expectation that a pregnant woman will
naturally "bond" with the child she is carrying collides with
her obligation to uphold her bond of trust[11] to the intended parents. This exposes the fact that maternal bonding may not be
as natural or automatic as is usually assumed, which disturbs
normative ideas of maternal bonding, maternal responsibility,
and, more widely, feminine behaviour. However, if a surrogate
mother does bond with the child she is carrying, she may find
it impossible to relinquish her to the intended parents, in which
case they remain childless and the child is left in an anomalous
position in a kinship system in which children are expected to
be brought up by their biogenetic parents. Thinking about maternal bonding from the perspective of surrogacy is therefore an
opportunity to examine and explore the nature, and the naturalness, of the maternal bond more carefully.

Erin, whose experience of pregnancy and birth I described
in the previous chapter, told me she felt attached to her daughter

from the moment she knew she was pregnant: "Psychologically, you're attached to this bundle of cells before it turns up. So arguably you're a mummy from the first day the pregnancy test produces two lines . . . and I think there is a bond and if you like, albeit imaginary, it's real, it's literal, but there is an element of sheer imagination and I think the bond [that] is created, that is built on and extended." Erin was also one of the people I knew during fieldwork who was most troubled by surrogacy. When I asked her if she thought a surrogate mother has a right to keep the baby if she decides she cannot hand her over to the intended parents, she said:

> Certainly, hundred percent, hundred percent. That's where my initial stomach-lurching fear at the start begins with all the people involved. I think that is a great example of that fear borne out, really. Such risks. I mean, I think there is a nine-month-long risk for a couple paying or involved in a surrogacy agreement . . . alright, there might be judgements that could be made about the whole situation, but I don't think there should be any negative judgement allotted to somebody changing their mind. And I think, yeah, that's where I find issues, how would that be if she wasn't brave enough to change her mind, risk [living] her whole life without her biological child and [then] a number of people are damaged? At the same time, I would feel gut-wrenchingly awful for two people that have grown attached to pictures on scans, have . . . emotionally as well as financially maybe invested in, you know, "their baby," which they see as their baby, and that's snatched from them at the very last [moment]. So I have great sympathy for them, but I think the mother concerned there, or the provider of the surrogate, has the right to change their mind at any time. And . . . that's nobody's right to judge.

Willow agreed with Erin that a surrogate mother had a right to keep the child if she changed her mind about relinquishing her to the intended parents. She explained, "I just have this feeling that it's their body and . . . you know, it's them that's been nurturing this baby and I just feel it's kind of theirs. Even if it hasn't, even if it's been another egg or what[ever], it's been theirs for the time it's been in them."

Quite a few people interpreted the "nightmare scenario" of a surrogate mother refusing to relinquish the child as a question of whether the child was, in fact, "hers."[12] This indicates their awareness that surrogacy has two forms: traditional surrogacy, in which the surrogate is inseminated with the intended father's sperm (so contributes her own egg), and gestational surrogacy, in which the surrogate is implanted with an embryo after the intended father's sperm has fertilised the intended mother's egg in vitro. Nina said quite bluntly, "Well, it's not her baby, is it? . . . Biologically, it's not hers. I mean, she's [just] carried it." Notably, when talking about her own reproductive plans in the previous chapter, Nina emphasised the importance of experiencing pregnancy, yet in talking about surrogate motherhood here she sidelined gestation in order to make a judgement about who is *the* "biological" mother. Andrew also argued that a gestational surrogate would have a less valid claim to motherhood: "I think that, whilst the nine-month period is very, very important . . . if she doesn't have any genetic link and she's been aware from the first instance that it was almost a business relationship—and I'd imagine they'd sign contracts these days, anyway—I don't think I would grant custody [to the surrogate] if I were a judge in that situation."

Some time ago, Lee Drummond examined earlier forms of "mother surrogation," including the work of domestic nannies in raising and rearing middle- and upper-class English children. He showed that not only is there variation in motherhood between different cultures but even within English society the mother concept is, and has historically been, "internally inconsistent."[13] Traditional practices like nannying, fosterage, and wet-nursing split maternal roles between different women and brought financial reward into maternal labour; historically, "blood ties" have been emphasised or deemphasised for particular purposes and different aspects of motherhood have been more or less defined by physical or emotional nurturance.[14] Drummond's analysis reminds us that there is a long history of maternal labour being split between different women but also that perceptions of such practices depend on contemporary discourses and ethics. Wet-nursing became popular in the context of a particular classed division of labour, but it was also possible because the idea of maternal bonding had less salience at the time.

This historical contingency in how we think about maternal bonding is highly relevant to ART and particularly surrogacy, since people involved in using these technologies know that such "natural" phenomena need to be carefully managed in order to avoid multiple and competing claims to parenthood. Various anthropologists have shown that those involved in surrogacy arrangements use concepts like nature and maternity contingently in order to preserve the claims of intended parents and to place surrogacy within a more socially acceptable frame.[15] Charis Thompson has written about the "strategic naturalizing" of patients in infertility clinics in America. She describes the clinic as "a site where certain bases of kin differentiation are foregrounded and recrafted while others are minimized to make the couples who seek and pay for infertility treatment—the intended parents—come out through legitimate and intact chains of descent as the real parents."[16] As she says in relation to the cases she encountered in the field, surrogacy and egg donation expose the fact that there is an "absence of a unique biological ground for answering the question, 'who is the mother,'"[17] yet through creative and strategic mobilisation of the possible answers to this question, patients and clinicians were usually able to create compelling arguments for each particular case, which drew on both biological and cultural factors to preserve procreative intent, kinship claims, and gender identity.

As these examples show, when we discussed surrogacy, people in Spey Bay formulated and expressed their ideas about maternal bonding in surrogacy in different, and sometimes contradictory, ways compared to how they thought about it in relation to conventional parenting and their own experiences. With surrogacy, they appealed to the "natural" concept of the maternal bond as if it were stable, whilst deploying it creatively to make particular and partisan claims. Thus Erin and Willow expected a surrogate mother to form a bond with the child because the maternal bond arises naturally out of the embodied experience of pregnancy. According to this reasoning, it is logically difficult to refute either a traditional or gestational surrogate mother's claim to the child since, as Lauren put it, "I can't really imagine carrying a small alien in your stomach for nine months and *not* feeling attached to it" (original emphasis). Nina and Andrew, meanwhile, claimed that the maternal bond comes from genetic kinship, so it would be impossible to deny a traditional surrogate's claim to motherhood, whilst gestational surrogacy is acceptable as the intended mother's claim represents a more comfortable balance of both biological and social motherhood. In making these distinct claims, each set of people drew on the concept of the maternal bond as a natural, and therefore given, phenomenon.[18]

The question of whether a surrogate mother has a right to claim parental rights over the child she has gestated and given birth to is a legalistic one, as Andrew's comments about awarding custody suggest. Paul felt that a legal contract could preclude the formation of a bond between a surrogate mother and the child. He said, "I assume people would [sign a legal contract], because that's where it all, for me, could go pear-shaped, because human emotion would come in. I mean, [the surrogate mother] could get attached to the baby in the womb, even, and once she sees it, you know, everything's gonna kick in, biologically and emotional attachment, you know, it could be very tricky." The first recorded surrogacy contract in the United States was made in the late 1970s, arranged by the (in)famous American surrogacy "broker" Noel Keane,[19] but surrogacy contracts are legally unenforceable in the UK, which retains the legal principle of *mater semper certa est*, or in other words, that the woman who

gives birth to a child is her mother until and unless custody is re-
linquished by or removed from her. Britain has therefore experienced only a small number of legal cases concerning surrogacy.[20]

In chapter 2 I recounted Sophie's discomfort with making
a judgement about postmenopausal women using ART that
was not "right-on," and when we talked about this quandary
the next day she told me, "Sometimes I think there's what you
feel and what you think you should feel." On the question of
whether a surrogate should be allowed to keep the child if she
wanted to, she said she hoped that the surrogate mother and
intended parents would discuss this possibility beforehand to try
to prevent such a conflict from occurring, though she added that
she could understand why a surrogate might feel like she could
not give up the child, describing the maternal bond as "this feeling that you hear people talking about that must be so different
and so compelling." Both Sophie and her friend and colleague
Amy found that thinking about a surrogate mother fighting for
custody forced them to consider the tough ethical dilemmas of
surrogacy. Amy said:

> I think it's just a really hard decision for someone to make in
> the first place and it kind of makes me think that surrogate
> parenting is bad, because how do you know? How can you
> kind of have a child and then give it away and then maybe
> down the line you would change your mind, but I don't think
> you could really change your mind because I don't think it's
> fair on the people that have started bringing up the child.

Sophie finally decided that she thought a gestational surrogate would have less of a claim to keep the child. I asked Amy
whether she thought it would make a difference if the egg came
from the intended mother rather than the surrogate and she said:

> I don't know. 'Cause that's really hard, 'cause if it's not the sur-
> rogate mother's egg and it's the other lady's egg, it just sounds
> horrible, talking about things like that being the property of

other people. I think that's when it gets complicated, 'cause the idea is really nice, that you're helping someone else have a child who can't have a child. But then, when we kind of talk about it as a piece of property, but then I guess that happens anyway, when parents split up—they argue over who's got custody over the children, so it's always gonna be an issue. Yeah, I don't know, it's very confusing!

Amy told me later that she found these questions difficult because she thought of herself as quite open-minded, but there were some things that we had talked about that made her have quite strong reactions. She said, "Sometimes I think if you can't have children, you can't, that's just nature," but it was clear that, like Sophie, she was not entirely comfortable with this judgement.

A Natural Feeling

In talking about surrogacy and maternal bonding, people commonly referred to feelings and emotion. They described emotions as physical, embodied experience and, as we saw in the last chapter, viewed the maternal bond as a feeling of attachment that compels a mother to respond to her child appropriately. The idea that a surrogate mother might decide to assert parental rights over the child she has carried for the intended parents was often expressed by people as a "change of mind," based on the assumption that feelings of attachment to the child might "kick in," causing her to feel that she was, after all, her mother.

Many believed that some process of psychological assessment would be appropriate before a surrogacy arrangement was set up, suggesting that counselling should be provided to the parties involved (but especially the surrogate mother), not only to provide emotional support but also as a means of vetting potential surrogates by weeding out those who are not emotionally fit for the role.[21] This idea that the assessment of a potential surrogate's psychological state may act as an appropriate measure of her suitability is commensurate with British clinical practice, as surrogates and intended parents are expected to attend repeated counselling sessions throughout the entire process.[22] By insisting that the surrogate be emotionally strong, in itself a rather labile measure, people implicitly set limits on surrogacy's availability.

People in Spey Bay agreed that "altruism," or feelings of love and sympathy towards the intended parents, was the best motivator for a surrogate mother, but the vast majority also believed that surrogate mothers are entitled to receive some payment for their service (see chapter 5). As Fenella Cannell[23] has pointed out, if surrogates can claim to be motivated by altruism towards the intended parents, even if they are also paid, then it may be easier to frame their behaviour as acceptable within wider cultural ideologies of femininity.[24] People assumed that if she were motivated by altruism then a surrogate would feel better about what she had done, because she could emphasise her motivation to help someone over the fact that she had "failed" to form a maternal bond and "given up" a child she had been pregnant with. For those who were in favour of surrogacy, the surrogate's "unnatural" relinquishing of the child she has carried would be obviated by her altruistic act of helping another, with whom she has formed, or has come to form, a bond of sisterhood or friendship that can replace the bond she might have formed with the child. In the British context, which prohibits paying the surrogate mother, this could also provide a "reward" for the surrogate mother.

As Catherine A. Lutz argued in her classic work, *Unnatural Emotions*, emotions confound the Cartesian splitting of mind and body because they are thought to originate in the mind but be felt in the body. Because they are seen in Western cultures as arising out of an individual's particular psyche, their social nature is rarely appreciated.[25] As Lutz argues, we need to recognise that emotions are as much an index of social relations as external manifestations of individuals' inner states.[26] Arlie Hochschild has described emotions as "signals" and "clues" to individuals' different perspectives and positions in the world. As she puts it, "Like hearing or seeing, feeling provides a useful set of clues in figuring out what is real."[27] As this case of people speculating about the emotional state and drives of surrogate mothers shows, the language of emotions is an important indicator of wider ethical values and "structures of feeling."[28] The example of surrogacy also reminds us that ideas about motive and human nature are gendered—women are expected to be naturally compelled towards altruism, and this is exemplified by motherhood and "maternal instinct."

Another important point made by Lutz is that emotions are strongly associated with nature and biology, which makes them appear given and inescapable. Here, when people talked about the "emotional strength" required of a surrogate mother, they were not only connecting mind and body through the language of emotions but also talking about nature. The concerns people expressed to me about the consequences of a surrogate forming a bond with the child and about her emotional state, particularly at the moment of postpartum handover, show the cultural and moral significance of this defining act in the surrogacy arrangement. Surrogacy is troubling because the surrogate is expected to resist a natural feeling that is supposed to be so strong and compelling that refuting it would be emotionally damaging.

Sophie described the gap between her own feelings about some forms of ART and what she thought were the correct feeling rules[29] according to her politics as "what you feel and what you think you should feel." As this suggests, emotions not only may signal a person's particular psychological makeup or subject position but also may be a base from which to form opinions and to work out what is right or good. In the debates that surround surrogacy, norms of motherhood, femininity, and kinship become, according to Strathern, "literalised,"[30] by which she means they are exposed to active attention, which can have the effect of making them seem less certain because they appear made rather than given. The ethical dilemmas provoked by surrogacy demonstrate that motherhood is heavily laden with moral values that inscribe expectations for proper behaviour and relationships and that are articulated in the language of nature, biology, and embodied feeling. Any challenge to maternal bonding, like the relinquishing of a child by a surrogate mother, seems to represent a threat to our most basic relationship and source of identity. For people in Spey Bay, the surrogate mother epitomised the anomalous and ethically fraught nature of surrogacy, and talking about her "unnatural" act of rejecting a child she had borne made their ideas about maternal bonding and motherhood explicit. But whilst surrogacy seems on the one hand to challenge fundamental values and axioms of kinship and parenting, it also provokes people to reproduce normative ideas about the nature and ethic of motherhood.

"A Sort of Community Thing"?

Whilst community has not typically been foregrounded in public representations of ART, it is important in these debates since they act as an arena in which a group of people deliberates about who they are and what they stand for. In enacting regulation of ART in both the United States and UK, the "plight of the infertile couple" has been a recurring trope, with advocates of the technologies casting the public, policymakers, researchers, and clinicians as the wider community who can help them to have children—or as the only ones stopping them.[31] As Michael Mulkay has shown, convincing politicians and the public that ART is intended for the public good of helping infertile couples have children and not about allowing scientists to "play god" was key to securing eventual support for the Human Fertilisation and Embryology Act, which provides the legal framework for ART and embryological research in the UK.[32]

When talking about reproduction, people in Spey Bay made repeated reference to an ethical framework that is not only about committing a good act for the sake of another individual but also about nurturing existing relationships and even building community. Ethnographic accounts of Britain have been characterised by a focus on community, so it should not be particularly surprising that people in Spey Bay were explicit about the importance of this fragile but viscous entity in their lives and aspirations for the future. In their influential forays into British village life—in the Shetland Isles and the southeastern English county of Essex, respectively—both Anthony Cohen[33] and Marilyn Strathern[34] deftly depict the minute differences that culminate in the making and unmaking of boundaries that are key to both community and belonging.[35] What they show in particular is that people can draw on different elements with more or less relevance to themselves in claiming belonging, from kinship to profession to club membership to shared beliefs.[36] These and other ethnographies of Britain show the importance of work, effort, and shared ideas in making community.

People's ideas about the ethics of surrogacy reveal much about maternal bonding but also about the status of market values in British culture,[37] including beliefs about motive and human nature, the ability of money to taint social relations, ideas about proper forms of work, and the importance of ethical values in structuring communities. In the next chapter I will return to people's ideas about payment for bodily and reproductive substances and services, including the distinction between altruistic and commercial surrogacy, which was in fact quite blurry for people in Spey Bay. As I have suggested in preceding chapters, for people in Spey Bay, "altruism" is a fundamental ethic that should motivate human relationships and that can provide the basis for building belonging and community, and it is highly relevant to the charitable work of the wildlife centre and other forms of ethical labour. In this section, I will probe a little deeper into what people meant by altruism in surrogacy. Like discussions about commercialisation and commodification in reproduction, people's ideas about altruism are vital in the stories they tell about who they are as ethical individuals—and communities.

IVF and, to a certain extent, donor conception are well on the way to becoming normalised in the UK, but there has been a lively debate about ART and embryological research since work on IVF began, which people in Spey Bay were well aware of. Although initial reactions to IVF and the birth of Louise Brown were largely positive, the length of time it took for legal regulation to be developed reflects how fundamentally these technologies shook common assumptions about the nature of human life, the propriety of scientific research, and the responsibilities of clinicians towards the communities in which they work.[38] During the parliamentary debates that led to the eventual legal regulation of ART and embryo research, many politicians and public commentators, including those strongly in favour of ART, saw surrogacy as one of the most troubling forms of ART, and the government's committee of inquiry led by Mary Warnock, most of whose recommendations made it onto the statute books intact, expressed deep-seated concerns about surrogacy.[39]

The legal regulation of surrogacy was given priority over other forms of ART, with the Surrogacy Arrangements Act (1985) being passed five years before the Human Fertilisation and Embryology Act (1990).[40] This was largely done to prevent any profit-making surrogacy agencies like the one that had recruited Kim Cotton from taking advantage of the legal vacuum to establish themselves in the country. The speed with which it was enacted probably reflected the fact that Cotton was already pregnant and that the agency that had recruited her had promised to set up surrogacy arrangements with more women shortly.[41] This haste also reflects the special anxieties that surrogacy provokes, and continues to provoke. The Human Fertilisation and Embryology Act was updated in 2008, though the overarching spirit of the Warnock Committee, which had informed the original act eighteen years earlier, prevailed. This update did make one relatively radical, if overdue, change, which was to remove the "need for a father" clause, thereby (at least in principle) enabling people to access ART whatever their sexuality or marital status. It also allowed for same-sex and unmarried parents to have access to surrogacy by permitting them to apply for Parental Orders, thus aligning the availability of surrogacy with other forms of donor conception. Otherwise, the law on surrogacy is largely unchanged since 1985 and surrogacy continues to provoke cultural and ethical unease in the UK. Public and media attention has in the last few years shifted towards the transnational surrogacy industry, especially in India, and the media are still quick to report on cases of surrogacy gone wrong, such as the Baby Gammy case in Thailand.

The Surrogacy Arrangements Act and the original 1990 Human Fertilisation and Embryology Act were both thought by policymakers to reflect public opinion, based on the media outcry about the Kim Cotton case and the deliberations of the Warnock Committee, respectively. They were intended to allow only new forms of technological assistance to human reproduction that were acceptable to the public conscience. The Surrogacy Arrangements Act essentially enshrines "altruistic surrogacy," in which any vestiges of a commercial transaction are eliminated, as the acceptable version of surrogacy in the UK. The maximum penalty for breaking section 2 of the act, negotiating surrogacy arrangements on a commercial basis, is three months in prison. In surrogacy arrangements, the intended parents have to apply for a Parental Order shortly after the child's birth (three weeks in the case of Scotland and six weeks in England, Wales, and Northern Ireland),[42] which transfers parental rights and custody to them from the surrogate mother, who, as noted earlier, is the prima facie mother in British law. The law prohibits the granting of Parental Orders to intended parents who have given surrogates more than "reasonable expenses." However, the act does not establish what is "reasonable," so, even in the law, the distinction between altruistic and commercial surrogacy is, in fact, a grey area and there is evidence that there have been "commercial" surrogacy arrangements in the UK that have not been prosecuted.[43]

In Helena Ragoné's foundational study of commercial surrogacy in America, the surrogates claimed that, although they were paid, they were motivated by altruism,[44] and the agents in her study found gift rhetoric invaluable in recruiting surrogates.[45]

Ragoné's findings complicate assumed dichotomies between commercial and altruistic surrogacy, as the "altruistic" gift becomes entangled in what is also a commercial exchange. "Pure" altruism is a cultural ideal, but real-life decisions by particular individuals will necessarily entail a complex mixture of motives that may be construed as "altruistic" or "selfish" according to when, where, and by whom such assessments are made. Whilst apparently aimed at the common good, purely altruistic or self-sacrificial actions, meanwhile, may be excessive and therefore antisocial;[46] in his germinal account of the gift, Marcel Mauss pointed out that gift exchange reproduces hierarchy, expresses aggression, and creates bonds of obligation.[47]

The model of surrogacy favoured by most people in Spey Bay was, broadly speaking, "altruistic," although in talking about altruism they tended to be more focused on the motives of the parties to a surrogacy arrangement (and in particular the surrogate mother) than on the spectre of profit-making surrogacy agencies. Rather than a supererogatory model of altruism in which one woman selflessly acts as a surrogate to help another woman out of compassion, their conception of altruism was much more focused on the idea of fostering community values.

Nina said she had heard media stories about surrogacy in which surrogates had been "taken advantage of" and she thought that "getting a stranger to be a surrogate for you would be very weird." She explained, "You have to keep it within your circle and the people you know or else . . . that's when it becomes a bit of a moral issue, for me. And I think [then] there'd be less chance of the end result not being right, as in someone keeping the baby and not actually giving it to the [intended] parents." Sophie made a similar point, saying that she did not like the idea of surrogacy as "a business transaction." Instead, she said, "I *do* like the idea of it as a sort of community thing and a family or a community caring for each other and trying to help out" (original emphasis).

Nina and Sophie's comments, which are illustrative of others', show their belief that "altruism" is the best reason for acting as a surrogate mother but also what they understand by altruism. For them altruistic surrogacy is an offer of support and assistance to known others that implies sympathy and mutual support; a means of preventing exploitation; knowledge between parties that ensures that obligations are fulfilled; and something that creates community, which is about "caring for each other and trying to help out." We also see what it is not: specifically, "taking advantage" of others and a "business transaction."

I asked Andrew what he thought would make someone want to become a surrogate mother, and he said that unless she was a "professional" surrogate mother who was motivated by money, then he could only really imagine her being motivated by an existing relationship with the intended parents. He said he thought the motivation would be "the actual knowledge of the people who are involved and wanting to help the relationship that's already there" out of "willingness" and "love" for the intended parents.

A couple of people told me that they had thought about acting as surrogate mothers themselves. Charlotte had a friend who had been diagnosed with spinal problems that meant she might not be able to carry a child to term, and she had told this friend that if she wanted to have children in the future she would consider acting as a surrogate for her. As she told me this story as we were rearranging stock in the wildlife centre shop one day, she did confess that she was relieved that her offer had never been taken up, which no doubt only increased when she became aware of her own potentially impaired fertility a few months later.

Lizzy volunteered at the wildlife centre on the weekends alongside studying for her Highers[48] and lived in a nearby town with her parents, who had migrated from England. She thought it would be a good idea for me to speak to her friend Alex, as she had offered to act as a surrogate mother for a gay mutual friend of theirs if he wanted to have children in the future. Unfortunately I never had the opportunity to meet Alex in person, but we did correspond by email and she told me her thoughts about surrogacy. She said:

I wouldn't consider being an anonymous surrogate. It would only be a consideration if it were for someone I knew very well that needed help. That way I would know what kind of a family the child would be going into, as well as I think it would make the whole experience easier, as in that situation you would not be thinking that you are having to give your baby away to a couple, it would be more of a case of knowing that you are really helping someone you care about and you can be excited for them having their baby and it just happens to be that it's through you. Also, you would be able to keep in touch and that would let the child know where they came from.

In this quote, Alex talks explicitly about knowledge four times, encompassing and addressing a number of concerns that she has about surrogacy. Knowledge here seems to stand for context. It also stands for trust, identification (in specific contrast to anonymity), the needs of others, and the promise of continuing future relationships. By focusing on knowledge, she separates out the act of giving up the child from that of "helping someone you care about." This rerouting means that she could see herself simply as a means "through" which their needs are fulfilled rather than as someone who has given a baby away. The idea of helping someone you know grounds her claim that surrogacy can be socially and morally acceptable. In Alex's formulation, "your" (the surrogate mother's) baby becomes "their" (the intended parents') baby. This not only reorients attention away from the means of the surrogacy arrangement (the surrogate mother) towards the end (the child) but also implies that thinking of others is a sufficient motivation for doing something.

Whilst Alex recognised that a surrogate mother may inevitably feel some attachment to the child, she believed that she should try and resist this in order to uphold her side of the surrogacy agreement. This anticipates the realities of commercial surrogacy arrangements as described by Helena Ragoné: "By focusing upon her relationship to the adoptive mother, in particular, to the idea that she is giving the adoptive mother a child, the surrogate shifts the emphasis away from her relationship to the father vis-à-vis the child and from the perception that she will be 'giving the baby away.'"[49] Ragoné concludes that this focus allows for the surrogate's actions to be cast "in a more socially acceptable light."[50] It also enables the arrangement to run "successfully," that is, to ensure that the child ends up with the intended parents, which further adds to surrogacy's public acceptability.

Alex was clearly uninterested in acting as an anonymous[51] surrogate, and one reason for this is to know "what kind of a family" the child would be raised in. In her study of anonymous British ova donors, Monica Konrad found that many donors, despite wishing to remain anonymous to the recipients of their eggs and unconnected to any resulting children, expressed a profound interest in the results of their donations, and specifically whether their "gift" had resulted in any live births.[52] As Konrad suggests, this complicates commonplace assumptions about both gifts and anonymity and the kind of sociality that they enact. Alex and others made the assumption that altruistic surrogacy is about helping *known* others. This suggests an inability to conceive of a scenario in which a surrogate or donor would be willing to go through the pain, inconvenience, potential stigma, and kinship ramifications of surrogacy or donation without some prior relationship of reciprocity, obligation, or love. People in Spey Bay were clear about the significance of knowledge in reproduction. It is important to know what kind of world a child will be born into, to know how parents are related to their children, and to know whether relationships will last, but knowledge is also important in terms of enabling ethical judgements because it allows for cases to be judged in context.

Context

How do you study reproduction and ART in the context of people's everyday lives? Surrogacy, like other ART, has typically been studied by social scientists in infertility clinics and surrogacy agencies and from the point of view of those using this reproductive technology. This move comes out of the laudable intention of early feminist scholars of science to find out what the experience of ART was like for those personally involved, which is of course vital to our understanding of them and the ways in which they are taken up. This approach does, however, need to be balanced with better understandings of what those who are not personally involved in these technologies, but who are exposed to them through media, public debate, government policies, and increasing research and development, think and feel about them. What can get lost in the attempt to pin down ethical principles and to codify legal regulations is the ambivalence, "strategic naturalizing,"[53] and creativity that ART inevitably seem to provoke.

When I was talking to people in Spey Bay, I was particularly struck by two discrepancies between what they thought about surrogacy and what I had expected they might think based on my knowledge of national public debates. One was the openness many people had to payment for surrogate mothers, which I discuss in the next chapter, and the other was the assumption a number of people made that surrogacy contracts would, and should, be legally enforceable. By assuming that surrogacy cases could be settled in court, Paul, for example, treated the legal system as a higher authority that could provide ultimate judgement about who is a child's mother, informed by an apparently accurate recognition of natural maternity. But his assumption—which was by no means unique to him—was out of sync with British law, which renders surrogacy contracts void and prioritises gestational experience over any contractual agreement. These differences in how people in Spey Bay thought about surrogacy are interesting precisely because the law is aimed at reflecting public feeling and the Warnock Report was, as a committee of inquiry, based on evidence collected from a range of interest groups, including medical researchers and clinicians, royal colleges, church groups, social workers, disability charities, "pro-life" groups, health authorities, and campaigners for women's health, as well as nearly seven hundred letters and submissions from the public. The Warnock Report sought to represent social consensus and bioethical principles on ART, and Mary Warnock has been candid about the pragmatism that underlay her own approach in steering her committee's recommendations.[54]

Researchers who work on ART have found over and again that one of the main reactions these technologies provoke is ambivalence. Ambivalence was evident in Amy's equivocation about the ethics of surrogacy, which she tried to comprehend in comparison with shared custody between divorced parents, and in Nina's contrasting comments about the importance of experiencing pregnancy in motherhood and the irrelevance of gestational experience to a surrogate mother's right to claim custody of the child she has carried in a surrogacy arrangement. The ambivalence that ART provoke is both an expression of and a reaction to the fact that these technologies are an attempt to assist nature (epitomised in the natural desire to have children of one's own and the natural process of sexual reproduction), and thereby conserve norms of kinship and sexuality, but which, by their substitutive and technological nature, cannot help but alter or subvert those very norms.

//

Following the Highland Council hearing I attended with Sophie, an Environmental Impact Assessment (EIA) was carried out on the Whiteness Head development and it was given the green light to go ahead in 2007. In fact, this never happened, and in 2012 another EIA took place, this time with a view to developing the site into a manufacturing and port facility for the construction of wind turbines. In January 2014, the Highland Council granted planning permission to develop the site accordingly. On the surface, wind farms—like any other source of renewable energy—seem incontrovertibly good for anyone with an interest in preventing climate change, but for those concerned about cetacean conservation, they provoke a great deal of ethical ambivalence. As with any sort of coastal construction, the noise caused by digging, building, and moving earth and metal around in order to establish the farms can interfere with marine mammals' ability to use echolocation to navigate, hunt, and find other members of their species. If the wind turbine plant goes ahead at Whiteness Head, it will threaten the Moray Firth dolphins, porpoises, and whales not only as it is built and developed itself but also in the products they will be producing there, the wind turbines. But then, perhaps it is a little churlish to overlook the commitment to renewable energy and environmental protection of industry and government that the plant also represents. Perhaps, in other words, it is worth risking the safety of a few dolphins in order to reduce humans' dependency on fossil fuels. Perhaps, in some form or another, nature will prove resilient after all.

Conclusion

Thinking about motherhood provoked people in Spey Bay to think about bonding. As the case of surrogacy indicates, bonding is a complex phenomenon that needs to be cultivated with care—this is especially so when it happens in ways that are not in line with natural expectations. Although surrogacy challenges the natural concept of the maternal bond and forces people into using nature in creative and strategic ways to account for it, its naturalness remained unquestioned. Concerns about motherhood often reflect wider social, political, and moral anxieties. In recent decades, people from across the political spectrum have publicly expressed concerns about motherhood in relation to changing gender roles, the well-being of children, the resilience of families, and demographic and social change.[55] As I noted earlier, the salience of certain aspects of motherhood has shifted through history, reflecting the fact that parenting is never only about nature or kinship but also about class, morality, economics, and politics. In a context in which nature seems in so many ways to be threatened and in which people feel increasingly divorced from the natural world, it is not surprising that people in Spey Bay should cleave to nature for guidance in assessing reproductive ethics. Perhaps also a wider sense of being separated from nature, or that reproduction is becoming denaturalised, is one of the reasons why increasing numbers of people in the Western world are turning to ART to create children "of their own" rather than adopting, co-parenting, or embracing childlessness.

Along with concerns about drifting away from nature, there is public concern in the UK about becoming too individualistic and too materialistic—or, to put it another way, less socially bonded. In this chapter, I have drawn attention to the salience of ideas of community in reproductive ethics. This was explicit in many of the responses from people in Spey Bay, which made it clear that how we deal with ART and reproduction more generally says something about who we are, not only as individuals but also as a local or national community. The idea of community is also relevant in that the regulation of surrogacy and ART in the UK is supposed to reflect public opinion, or a moral community. As this suggests, reproductive ethics are not only about individuals' or couples' private decisions about whether and how to have children but also about what is socially, morally, and legally acceptable to the larger community. Altruistic surrogacy means different things to different individuals and its practice is evidently less clear-cut than the law might imply, yet enshrining it in law as the British model of surrogacy gives an important message about the UK and its approach to reproduction, ethics, nature, women, and the family.

// *The Sperm Whale's Teeth Revisited*

Let me return briefly to the crime scene of the prologue. I went back later that December Friday to see the whale's body again. Hurrying with trepidation and excitement, I came up to the bank of sand dunes that overlooked its sandy open grave where I had stood, awestruck, that morning. This wretched, ransacked body, so lifeless a few hours earlier, was moving. Silenced by confusion and shock then laughing with a mixture of revulsion and relief at this magic realist sight, I understood my mistake. The tide had come in so that the water was just high enough to almost cover the whale but not enough to wash it away, so that it remained tethered to the beach by its own weight, whilst its tail and what remained of its head swayed and crashed like a circus animal trying to break free from its cage.

Diving a little deeper into this story, by following the teeth back to the days in which they washed up on the beach, reveals that this was no simple marine mammal morality tale. We had learned of the beaching on a Thursday evening and resolved to go and see it early the next morning before it had started to decompose or had been removed. In planning the trip, I was surprised to hear my friends from Spey Bay joking about slipping a pair of pliers into their pockets and extracting one of the teeth to sell on the Internet or to display in the wildlife centre in order to attract more visitors. When we came upon the scene, this mercenary banter quickly dissipated and was replaced by a sombre reverence befitting the atmosphere of mourning.

Later that day, when we had returned from Roseisle, they self-consciously made fun of themselves for ever entertaining the idea, however ironic its intention, that they could have had the stomach for looting the whale's teeth themselves. For a moment, these people who care so deeply about the plight of endangered cetaceans considered marine grave robbing. But, brought up short by the negative space where a jaw should have been, they were quick to realise this theft was unpalatable, though evidently not entirely immoral. The real tragedy for them, I believe, was not the extraction of the whale's body parts but its death, and the liability for that lay elsewhere, on the consciences of anonymous, as opposed to simply unknown, others: unscrupulous businesses exploiting the sea's resources and robbing this whale of its food, habitat, and life.

The wildlife crime officer had told us, during the local action group meeting in which he discussed the case, that the family who had apparently taken the jaw "act as if they are the local lairds." The lairds of Scotland may have been the traditional rulers, but they are also popularly associated with the inequalities of a feudal aristocracy, which does not fit with Scotland's contemporary image of itself as a place founded on meritocracy and egalitarianism. For most, lairds are less figures of traditional authority and more signifiers of oppression and hardship for ordinary people. In making this comparison, then, the wildlife crime officer—a representative of modern state power but also of the belief that protection of the natural world should be enshrined in law—criticised the putative thieves for both claiming undeserved privilege and exploiting natural resources.

From the point it was discovered stranded on Roseisle beach, the whale's body posed a practical problem in the tacit recognition that, whatever grief it provoked, like all corpses it would need to be disposed of. Options included using a controlled explosion to break it into more manageable pieces, a method that has been employed elsewhere including one case of a stranded orca on Spey Bay beach in the 1950s. Instead the local council removed the body to a rendering plant a few days later. The head was split into two parts, one delivered to the National Museum of Scotland in Edinburgh, the other to the wildlife centre in Spey Bay, with the intention that each would display their skeletons for visitors.

The wildlife centre also received the infamous jaw once the police had recovered it. Once again, conversation turned to the grotesque, faced with the pressing problem of how to deal with a decomposing cetacean's jaw in the absence of any specialist equipment or expertise for such a situation. Eventually the staff at the wildlife centre decided to leave it in a disused courtyard inside a metal drum filled with biological washing powder, which, over many months, eventually ate away the flesh and stripped the bones. The sperm whale's teeth remained a recurring subject in conversations as, with macabre bravado, they compared notes on how many times and in what state of decomposition they had seen them and on the strange journey they had taken to end up in Spey Bay.

Money Talks

The burden of responsibility placed on the
ethnographer is to acknowledge and make
unavoidable the engagement with alternatives that
is the grounds of moral and ethical action.

—Arthur Kleinman

"Put Your Sperm to Good Use"

Whilst eating dinner with Steve, Sophie, and Willow in a pub
one night, the conversation turned to sperm donation. In contrast to Jeanette Edwards's co-conversationalists in Lancashire,
who were coy about discussing ART in public arenas,[1] and the
stereotype that British people are uneasy talking about sexual
matters, many of the people I knew in Spey Bay were quite
comfortable with such discussions. ART did come up in conversation occasionally, partly in direct reference to my interest
but also in the course of conversations about families, friends,
and people's experiences of and plans for parenthood.

Steve was in his early thirties and worked in forestry and
tourism. When I first arrived in Spey Bay, he was sharing a house
with Sophie but moved out after buying a flat. Whilst he never
officially volunteered in the wildlife centre, he helped out on
many occasions and regularly attended social gatherings. Steve
rhetorically positioned himself as the "alpha male" of the group
in Spey Bay and frequently complained about being surrounded
by so many women, whom he often teased for talking about
whales and dolphins nonstop. He was also seen as someone who

took his environmental responsibilities very seriously and as a sensitive and loyal friend.

On this occasion, Sophie was teasing Steve about consuming pornography and asked him, "Why don't you put your sperm to good use by becoming a sperm donor?"

Steve turned to me and asked, "Could I could get paid for it?"

"You can get expenses," I said.

"What about for egg donors?" asked Willow.

As I responded, Sophie interjected with a sound of disapproval, then said, "It's funny, my immediate reaction there was that it's wrong to get paid for eggs but not for sperm, 'cause it's just sort of different, but I'm not sure why."

"Maybe it's to do with amounts, you know, like with fish, they have thousands of eggs and it's a certain amount," suggested Willow.

Sophie said, "I'm just trying to work out why there's a difference. I think maybe I think that an egg is more like a potential baby and the sperm is just something you add, like, you always think of the sperm coming in and fertilising the egg."

"So, would it be more like you were paying for a baby if you paid for an egg?" I asked. Sophie agreed and I then asked, "Do you think the difference has to do with the different processes of collection as well?" Steve and Sophie laughed.

"It might be a factor," admitted Sophie.

"Collecting sperm is definitely more fun than collecting eggs," said Steve.

"With egg collection, it's kind of dangerous, there's much more risk," concluded Willow.

In this conversation, sperm donation was portrayed as straightforward and comical, and therefore not problematically associated with payment, whilst egg donation was an emotive and onerous procedure that should not be rewarded with money. Whilst there are obvious differences between the physical experiences involved in sperm and egg collection, these distinctions also point to a gendered difference in what is fungible and what kind of "work" or "donation" can be appropriately rewarded with payment.[2] Specifically, egg donation is "dangerous" not only in terms of the risks of a surgical procedure but also because if women are paid for elements of their (potential) maternity they are symbolically rejecting the cultural model that posits mothers as naturally altruistic and as aspiring towards motherhood.

This conversation occurred in a pub in Findhorn, a village west of Spey Bay on the Moray Firth coast, which is also home to a Christian eco-community. The Findhorn community is on the outskirts of Findhorn village and consists of various types of alternative housing from state-of-the-art eco-homes to dwellings repurposed from whisky fermentation vats to caravans and prefabs. The main entrance to the site is off the road that leads into Findhorn village, with a shop that sells produce from their gardens as well as other "ethical" products, a car park, a visitor information hut, and, beyond that, a café and hall that is used for public events such as film screenings as well as private meetings amongst residents. The village of Findhorn has a spectacular sandy beach, pretty stone houses, and a handful of good places to eat and I visited it with people from Spey Bay many times. Whilst they recognised that they shared many of the principles of the Findhorn community and appreciated their aims, they were also a little uncomfortable with the idea of self-consciously building an exclusive community and so tended to associate themselves with the village more than with the eco-community.

As their differing loyalties to the parallel communities in Findhorn suggest, people in Spey Bay have not explicitly rejected capitalist modes of work by going "back to the land" or living "off grid," and they reject more extreme or utopian models of community building in favour of a more pragmatic and balanced approach to living a good life. They are canny in the way that they make good lives. The word "canny" comes from *can*, which in sixteenth-century Scotland meant "know" (and presumably is closely related to the northeast Scottish *ken*). The dictionary definition of canny is "having or showing shrewdness

and good judgement, especially in money or business matters."[3]
In Scotland and northeast England, it has another inflection—
describing someone as canny can be a compliment about their
pleasantness. Knowledge, judgement, and being nice to others
are entwined in this word, so it is apt in describing how people
in Spey Bay handle money in relation to making good lives.

People in Spey Bay do not think of money as inherently corrupting but hold individuals responsible for their own decisions
about how they make and spend it. In this chapter, I will describe their thoughts about the donation of bodily substances
and services in more detail, in order to extend the discussion
of the connections between community values and reproductive ethics, as well as to explore the circulation and meanings
of money in their personal and professional lives. In doing so,
I will return to questions about the contextual nature of ethics
and the broad significance of reproduction in everyday life.

"Selling Your Body for Nine Months"?

I mentioned Sophie Day's work on London sex workers in
chapter 1 not only because the contrast between charity work
and sex work, as two forms of female-dominated labour, is
thought provoking but also because many commentators, feminist scholars, and bioethicists have, in arguing against commercial surrogacy,[4] drawn an analogy between surrogacy and
sex work. This parallel also occurred, without my prompting,
to a few people in Spey Bay when we talked about surrogacy.
For example, Andrew said, "I certainly don't agree with people
paying for surrogates, or ladies selling themselves. It's a much
larger scale of prostitution in a way, I guess, selling your body
for nine months rather than a night." Richard did not straight-
forwardly object to prostitution or commercial surrogacy on
moral grounds but was, instead, concerned for the welfare of
the women involved and their likely exploitation. When I talked
with him about commercial surrogacy, he asked rhetorically, "A

country that can't even regulate prostitution properly without there still being some harm being done to the women, can it handle surrogacy?" Making a connection between commercial surrogacy and prostitution is not the same as saying that surrogate mothers are prostitutes, but it does suggest that there is some overlap between them and thereby sets up an association between surrogacy and the kind of moral, and economic, unease that sex work provokes. Andrew used this connection to express his fears about the commodification of women's bodies, whilst Richard used it to convey his concern about the endemic exploitation of women.

Much of the anticommercial surrogacy polemic of the late twentieth century is based on a model in which humans are properly "above" the market sphere and in which certain body parts and services should be kept separate from the commercial world. Anthropologists have identified this model as itself an artefact of capitalist society.[5] One key feature of this polemic is the "slippery slope" argument, that allowing money into surrogacy arrangements breaks down the barriers around those things, like blood, sex, and babies, that are considered properly outside the realm of commodity exchange, rapidly leading to a situation in which everything is commodifiable and every exchange is a financial transaction. Viviana Zelizer has noted a tendency amongst economic theorists to assume that money has the capacity to penetrate all spheres of life and that once it does so, emotional and social ties will be eclipsed by rational self-interest and the pursuit of material gain.[6] This way of thinking is also expressed in the section on surrogacy in the Warnock Report, which says: "That people should treat others as a means to their own ends, however desirable the consequences, must always be liable to moral objection. Such treatment of one person by another becomes positively exploitative when financial interests are involved."[7]

Paul told me that his views on commercial surrogacy had changed somewhat since he first heard of it but that he still found it problematic. He told me, "I just thought it was another example of people making money out of something, using something as a baby machine. That's the way I saw it at first." But he said that his views have shifted and that he could see an argument for reimbursing a surrogate's expenses. He explained, "I don't see that it's necessarily morally wrong. I just still think it's a bit bizarre doing something like that for money, as a service. If it was done by somebody you knew or somebody doing it for nothing, then it would seem better somehow, more acceptable to help that person."

Lauren felt that surrogates should receive payment to cover their costs plus "some amount of money for their 'efforts.'" But she was concerned about exploitation and said, "If you're paying a [surrogate] mother £5 million for nine months, that's going to put a lot of pressure on people to make that choice, not because they are comfortable with it, but because they need the money." Many people agreed with Lauren that surrogate mothers should receive some compensation for the time they are pregnant, especially if it means they have to stop working, though they also felt this would be difficult to regulate and were wary of suggesting a maximum amount of compensation. Nina argued that the intended parents should help the surrogate with any out-of-pocket costs related to the pregnancy but qualified this with characteristic frankness, saying, "I think paying a fee to get a life is just too much. I think it's morally wrong and a bit sick." Revulsion at the idea of "baby-selling" is the cornerstone of regulation against commercial surrogacy, and for some, commercial surrogacy necessarily implies buying a life rather than paying a woman for her reproductive labour.

Erin was more outspoken than anyone in her condemnation of commercial surrogacy. She said, "I think where there's the exchange of human beings and money . . . it takes us back to the Dark Ages. It takes us, you begin to question: did Wilberforce do anything for the human race? You question where our morals are at in the twenty-first century." Erin's argument is framed by a certain idea of progress, in which milestones like the abolition of slavery mark the progress of human civilisation.

The "Dark Ages" is in the British idiom a time of archetypal moral corruption compared to the apparently morally enlightened twenty-first century in which slavery is seen as very wrong. This analogy, as well as making it clear that Erin is deeply concerned about surrogate mothers being exploited and commodified, reminds us that the commodification of people is not a new phenomenon.[8] Surrogacy is often likened to both slavery and prostitution in public discourse, but of course both comparisons are, like any other form of merographic thinking, ambiguous—commercial surrogates are "like" slaves in that their bodies, or a function of their bodies, are commodified and because they cannot escape their "bondage" once they are pregnant, whilst altruistic surrogates could be seen as slaves as they are not paid for the "work" they do.

For Erin, the commodification of babies and women's bodies that commercial surrogacy represents was a cause for real anxiety, which she suggested would have dire consequences for the wider society. She said, "There's something quite emotionally—not to use a pun, but—barren about, barbaric, about, you know, handing over money and somebody walks off with a child." Her view that allowing money into the creation of human life negates the fecund potential of assisted conception by corrupting civilisation and rendering society "barren" resonates strongly with people's fears about ART leading to human endangerment that I discussed in chapter 2. Again, it shows that endangerment, the inability to produce future generations, is the ultimate threat that anyone faces and the belief that human actions can make endangerment more likely. Erin was also concerned about price: "You can't put a price on human life. What message are we giving to that child? You know, what, is one child worth [£]15,000, another worth [£]20,000? It's ludicrous, and I can't morally justify that situation to myself."

Andrew, like most others, believed that it was justified to give surrogate mothers some compensation. I asked him if he was concerned about payment changing the motivations of the parties in a surrogacy arrangement, and he said, "I think it would certainly change the motivations of the surrogate. I don't think it would change the motivation of the parents-to-be. . . . Well, I guess, if an egg and sperm match, do you choose the prettiest surrogate? Do you pay more for one with big breasts?! How does it work?"[9] Although Andrew was clearly a lot more sympathetic to commercial surrogacy than was Erin, he was, as his rhetorical question about pricing up a surrogate mother suggests, also concerned about the commodification of people and body parts that it might provoke.

Igor Kopytoff has shown that commodification is a process of becoming rather than being and that "the only time when the commodity status of a thing is beyond question is the moment of actual exchange."[10] As he said, "The same thing may, at the same time, be seen as a commodity by one person and as something else by another. Such shifts and differences in whether and when a thing is a commodity reveal a moral economy that stands behind the objective economy of visible transactions."[11] People in Spey Bay were concerned that a certain level of payment would tip a surrogacy arrangement over into unethical practices of exploitation and bodily commodification. Though no one suggested a specific amount, or "price," at which this might happen, the main anxiety seemed to be that there was a tipping point at which money could become the motivating factor for the surrogate mother. Thus people's fears about exploitation were not only about surrogate mothers being mistreated by the intended parents or a surrogacy agency but also about the surrogate mother's motive. They believed that surrogate mothers may be financially rewarded for their "efforts" but should not be primarily motivated by money. In contrast to the idea that money has a motivating force in itself, or that it can taint and colour social transactions, people in Spey Bay had a sense that, in financial transactions, it is the people involved in the transaction who have responsibility for the decisions they make.

Although Andrew would prefer that surrogacy be done according to an altruistic model, he recognised the argument for compensation, saying with a hint of irony in his voice, "It's like a job, having a job for nine months, I suppose." Lizzy told me, "It feels a bit wrong to have [the surrogate mother] being paid in a sense, as in a salary for a job, as it is much more than that. I would think that the couple who have asked the woman to carry the child will 'pay' the mother in their own way but then again what if they don't? Then I begin to think maybe some money should be put aside for the [surrogate] mother." Lizzy saw money as an insufficient, rather than corrupting, form of payment for surrogacy, but she also thought that recompensing the surrogate mother would be a way of caring for her.

Jenny said she would prefer that surrogacy occur between friends or family members based on ties of mutual support and was somewhat concerned about the potential for exploitation of women who acted as surrogates, but she suggested that the involvement of money in surrogacy arrangements was not necessarily immoral. Jenny was reflexive about the place of money in society. She remarked that although she is not a materialistic person herself, money is "the currency by which we measure a lot of things," and so she said about paying a surrogate mother, "I don't think it's necessarily a bad thing. I think it's valuing what somebody's doing for you in a very profound way."

If surrogacy can be conceptualised as being like a job in the efforts it entails and if money is generally an appropriate reward for work done or services rendered, then there is a clear argument for paying surrogate mothers. Importantly, these comments suggest there *is* room within the way that motherhood is conceptualised by people in Spey Bay for it to be associated with financial reward. It was noticeable in what they said to me that there was a meaningful distinction between payment and compensation for them but that it was far from clear where one stopped and the other began. Thinking about commercial surrogacy again shows the importance of context in knowing what is right or wrong in any particular case and therefore suggests the difficulty, and perhaps folly, of trying to draw up legislation based on a universalised model of reproductive ethics. The ethics of a particular situation are never fixed in advance, and the nuanced nature of these responses suggests that public and legal discourse does not do justice to the sophistication of people's attitudes and the complicated interstices of knowledge that they bring together when making ethical judgements.

Much of the public and bioethical revulsion against commercial surrogacy is based in a view of the world as split into the calculated, rational, profit-driven sphere of work and the warm, affective, and caring sphere of home, which makes any blurring of the boundary between the two seem inevitably exploitative. But this worldview is not only part of the fabric of capitalist ideology, it is also, as I noted in chapter 1, an increasingly anachronistic one in a twenty-first-century world of flexible, casualised, and precarious labour. As Melinda Cooper and Catherine Waldby write in their analysis of clinical labour, the "donation" of gametes, tissue, and gestational labour is not a marginal outlier of this post-Fordist economy but in fact closely entwined with it.[12] Since the 1970s, they write, "Domestic tasks, sexual services, care provision, and . . . the process of biological reproduction itself have migrated out of the private space of the family into the labor market and are now central to post-industrial accumulation strategies."[13] In this world, the sale of gametes and commercial surrogacy have flourished, reproducing stratifications of class, gender, and race whilst also entrenching forms of "work" that provide little protection from risk or long-term security for those providing their bodily tissues or reproductive labour. Whilst British law on gamete donation and surrogacy has always been explicitly aimed at preventing donation from becoming selling and surrogacy from becoming a paid service, recent increases in compensation rates for egg donors in the UK (a tripling from £250 to £750) and the increasing participation of British intended parents in the expanding transnational ART market belie this apparent moral purism.

Thicker than Water

Debates about reproductive technologies make our cultural beliefs and moral principles apparent. A strong strain of anti-Americanism was evident in the public revulsion at the Kim Cotton commercial surrogacy case,[14] which was set up by an American agency.[15] Resisting the penetration of the free market into private spheres of life is important in how British people represent themselves as a humane and civilised people.[16] America is often stereotyped by people in Britain as its more money-oriented and commercialised cousin, and in Kim Cotton's case, much polemic focused on rejecting the "American" ideas of women "renting" their wombs and couples "buying" babies.[17]

Given the provocative parallels between blood donation and the donation of reproductive substances and services, I asked people in Spey Bay what they thought about paid blood donation and whether they had donated blood themselves.[18] Their responses, once again, say much about the contingency of ethics as well as the close relationship between community and ethics. In his classic comparative study of blood donation systems, Richard Titmuss concluded that, overall, the "altruistic" model of blood donation as used in Britain is a healthier and more efficient basis for a transfusion service than the largely commercial one in place in the United States at the time.[19] Titmuss wrote that blood donation systems tell us "something about the quality of relationships and of human values prevailing in a society,"[20] and his belief that voluntary or "altruistic" donation is not only more efficient but also more moral is clear from his analysis.

In making these arguments, Titmuss drew on Marcel Mauss's classic theory of the gift, though, as a number of anthropologists have pointed out, his use of Mauss's work was partial. Richard Tutton has summarised some of these criticisms, including specifically the importance of obligation and reciprocity in Mauss's model of gift giving, which is largely passed over in Titmuss's depiction of the ideal type of the "voluntary community donor."[21] Tutton argues that anthropological theory on the gift and the gift-commodity opposition within the wider culture had "metaphorical resonance" for Titmuss in his theorisation of blood donation, in a context of wider debates about the values of community, altruism, and social equality—all of which Titmuss was keen to promote and which he felt the postwar welfare state embodied.[22] Tutton suggests that Titmuss's characterisation of the "gift" of voluntary blood donation should be read in this context—as a defence of the welfare state and as an attack on commercialism, which was in this instance signified by the American model of marketised private health care.[23] Ultimately it was also an argument about British values.

Generally speaking, people in Spey Bay would prefer for people not to be paid for donating blood, but they did perceive there to be a shortage of blood and so conceded that remuneration might be helpful in attracting more donors. People felt that, as with surrogacy or gamete donation, the best reason for giving blood is altruism. Some referred to a generalised altruism, like Alex, who argued, "I don't think that blood donors should be paid for donating as people should not need a cash incentive to help save people's lives." When I talked about it with Joanna, she referred to an earlier conversation I had had with her about voluntary work. When volunteering at the wildlife centre, she never accepts any of the expenses for lunch and travel costs she is entitled to because, she told me, it is her choice to work there and she "doesn't do it for the money." On blood donation, she said, "I wouldn't want to be paid for it. It's like what we said about volunteering—you volunteer to do something and then if you're getting paid for it you're not actually volunteering anymore. So no, I don't think people should." Lauren, who is American, made voluntary blood donations in the United States before she moved to Scotland. Whilst she could see an argument for reimbursing donors' expenses, she said that if people were able to "abuse" the system it would be a sign that "we've got very skewed community values and social values" but suggested that if money were used to educate people and promote donation, then it could instead "fund understanding and create a sense of community."

Andrew is both a blood donor and a registered organ donor. He seamlessly combined altruism and self-interest in explaining his reasons for donating blood: "I think you should do it because you think it's going to help other people and you might be in the position that you need it yourself, not because someone gives you a fiver to do it." Erin was similarly candid about why she gave blood: "You do it in the hope that, God, if you ever need a blood bag or . . . one of your loved one does, there's one there for them . . . we're all human beings and we're all in it together and we're all trying to help each other out. It's a humanistic principle." Giving blood is, according to this "humanist" model, an investment in the future, whether a general pool or your kin network. In this model, which seems to be based on an idea of social solidarity rather than supererogatory altruism, the distinction between altruism and self-interest is blurred: Erin and Andrew give blood because they feel it is a moral action that benefits other people *and* because it might benefit them or their family.

Historically, in the UK and elsewhere, blood has been seen as the metaphorical and literal carrier of kinship. Though we have absorbed genetics into our folk models of kinship and inheritance with alacrity, blood remains thick with meaning, and Janet Carsten found in her interviews with Scottish blood donors that many of them referred to kinship as both a motive for donating and a source of connection with other donors and recipients.[24] In terms of donation, blood seems to flow much more easily than gametes, despite the fact that they are all replaceable—bodies make new sperm and blood and most women's ovaries will produce far more eggs than they will ever need. Despite the thick meanings of blood—and of course they go far beyond the domain of kinship—giving blood is, ethically speaking, relatively unproblematic compared to gamete donation or surrogacy. Blood is thought of as much more partible from its original body largely because, unlike gametes and embryos, it does not seem to contain a (potential) new human being.

As with gamete donation and surrogacy, perceived motive was very important in how people in Spey Bay viewed the ethics

of paid blood donation. Erin said that if the NHS started offering £5 for blood donations it would be unlikely to make her
give more but that if they offered her £5 when she got there then
she would probably accept it. Erin did not have the same concerns about paid blood donation as she did about commercial
surrogacy. When I pointed this out to her, she explained that she
saw one as selling babies and the other as selling blood and that
these were two very different things: "A blood bag . . . doesn't
have a personality, it doesn't have a soul."

Like Erin, Paul thought that donating bodily substances
was very different from surrogacy. He told me, "I don't see
anything wrong with being paid to donate sperm" and joked
that, because of his age, "I don't think anyone would want mine
now, otherwise you'd have given me a nice little earner." He explained that donating blood or sperm for money "might just be
some way of making some money for people, and I don't see any
harm in that. But it's not the same as creating and developing a
human life. It's not the same at all, is it? Blood isn't the same as a
baby, there's a big difference there, you're talking about a human
being." Whilst both Erin and Paul were clear that there is a significant difference between bodily substances like blood and
sperm on the one hand and a "baby" on the other, it is notable
and somewhat surprising that neither of them referred to kinship in describing this difference, except in the very generalised
sense of shared humanity. This was also true in the pub conversation about sperm and egg donation that I described earlier.

Jenny had a similar viewpoint to that of her partner, Paul,
but, again, she was more reflexive than others about the relationship between ethical values and cultural identity. As we
drank herbal tea in their cottage, she told me about donating
blood in return for money when she was living in Greece in
her twenties and observed that blood donation is "promoted in
[British] culture, our very localised culture, as being an altruistic
action. I don't necessarily think that payment's offensive, but I
think we've promoted it in our society hitherto as an altruistic
thing." She said that she thought that egg donors, sperm donors,

and surrogate mothers should all have their costs reimbursed but noted again that because "creating a new life is imbued with high emotional and moral standards," people feel that it is better if such actions are made "for love of fellow mankind, rather than a straightforward financial transaction."

In talking about the ethics of blood donation, gamete donation, and surrogacy people in Spey Bay drew subtly different distinctions, using particular and competing logics. As Michael Lambek has said of the gift, the Maussian obligations to give, receive, and reciprocate the gift are "neither mechanical acts of rule-following nor simple or maximizing choices."[25] Instead, as in other ethical judgements, gift givers must weigh up and balance competing considerations and commitments. People's ideas about commercial and altruistic surrogacy as well as paid blood, egg, and sperm donation show this contingency in practice. It also echoes the strategic ways in which they discussed maternal bonding (see chapters 3 and 4). Attempts to define ethics or to use ethics as a basis for legislation are at odds with how ethics is experienced on an everyday basis because they erase the contingency that is characteristic of ethical reflection, judgement, and action. Reproduction is, as I stated in the introduction, enmeshed in wider ethical struggles. If we divorce it from its social, relational, economic, political, ecological, religious, or moral contexts, we are denaturing its meaning and overlooking the importance it has in everyday lives.

People in Spey Bay recognise that money is necessary for everyday life and that it is mixed in with affective ties. One clear example of how vital money is to everyday ethics in Spey Bay is fund-raising. The Adopt a Dolphin scheme is the financial backbone of the charity that runs the wildlife centre. Adopters pick a dolphin from a shortlist of Moray Firth dolphins, which are profiled in leaflets and on the charity's website with their name, sex, and "personality." Adopters sign up for a monthly standing order donation to the charity. At the time of the adoption they receive an information pack, including a soft toy dolphin and badge, and through the adoption period they continue to receive regular updates about the Moray Firth dolphins, cetaceans further afield, and the work of the charity. The soft toy dolphin of course adds to the anthropomorphism of dolphins that many staff members find problematic, but it also helps smooth over the fact that this is an act of cross-species gift giving. The programme is largely marketed at children, though it is usually paid for by adults. This relates to popular ideas about dolphins appealing to children and taps into the belief that adults should work to protect their children from human-made problems of climate change and species endangerment in the future that I discussed in chapter 2. Many of the new adoptions I observed in the wildlife centre were parents adopting dolphins on their children's behalf, though quite a few visitors to the centre were people who had adopted dolphins some time ago and had made a special trip to Spey Bay to try to spot "their" dolphin in the flesh.

The term "adoption" posits a kinship link between adopter and dolphin, implying a closer solidarity than between a mere cash donor and recipient and drawing attention away from the financial aspect of this transaction. The idiom of adoption helps to personalise and individualise the donation when, in fact, as with other charities with similar schemes, the money goes towards advocacy, events, projects, and running the charity's wildlife centres. Conservation charities rely on their causes' cultural, ethical, and economic value in order to help them. Dolphins and whales are charismatic megafauna[26] and conservation groups recognise that emphasising their benign and in some ways human-like nature helps secure financial and popular support for their cause, even if it provokes ethical ambivalence amongst themselves.

Jonathan Parry argues that in contemporary capitalist societies like the UK, charitable good works and disinterested giving are the counterparts to pure utility, resting on the idea that persons and things are separate.[27] As he says, "The ideology of a disinterested gift emerges in parallel with an ideology of purely interested exchange."[28] The same people who make "pure" gifts carry out financial transactions in their daily lives, but with the development and expansion of capitalism these different types of transactions come to be increasingly morally differentiated, so that gifts become laden with associations of altruism, love, and emotionality whilst economic exchanges come to be conceptualised as divorced from human emotion and characterised by rational calculation.

Despite the ideology of pure gift and pure commodity in capitalism, altruism, greed, exploitation, and commodification cannot be separated in people's thinking, discourse, or practice. Fund-raising for charity is, in one sense, a pragmatic recognition that helping any cause in a capitalist society relies on finance, but it also complicates these dichotomous relations between commodities and gifts. A donation of money to charity seems very much like a "pure gift," even if it is a gift of money and, by adopting a dolphin or putting money in a charity tin, donors are "buying" altruism, or good ethics. Charities have brands and in their marketing they capitalise on their causes' moral value whilst also cultivating affect in their potential supporters. Capitalist values, like any other values, may be called upon in flexible and contingent ways and will be weighed up against each other in making ethical decisions.

Making

Whilst I was a participant observer in Spey Bay, I found myself regularly making food. Having grown up with a particular set of beliefs about what work looks and feels like, I found it hard to adjust to the idea that hanging out with people counted as work whilst I was doing my fieldwork. One way in which I countered this was to keep busy with domestic tasks, which was also a way of reciprocating Sophie's hospitality. In Spey Bay, I grew small crops of salad and herbs in the front garden outside her house, I helped look after her chickens, I baked bread, and I cooked.

I mentioned the multiple sources and values that go into buying and making food in Spey Bay in the introduction. This was something I started to learn the first time I attended a barbecue in Spey Bay, not long after I had started volunteering there. The barbecue had not been planned in advance, but the mild weather suggested it and a number of staff members and volunteers enthusiastically agreed to stay on after work to spend the evening with their colleagues. We needed ingredients, though, and I readily volunteered to drive to the shops. I went to the nearest supermarket, rather than the local butcher, whose excellent produce I had yet to discover, and unthinkingly chose some meat that was in a three-for-the-price-of-two offer. I say unthinking, though perhaps it would be more accurate to say that rather than weighing up the ethics of the food's provenance, I was prioritising feeding as many people as possible. I was trying to be generous to my fellow guests rather than caring for the environment.

When I returned to Spey Bay with the meat and a few other items, no one said anything critical about my choices (though they did not say anything positive, either), and indeed once the meat was removed from its plastic casing and was cooking on the barbecue, it would have been hard to tell where it was from anyway. But by observing the ways in which others sourced their food and participating in conversations about food ethics as I spent more time at Spey Bay and came to know people better, I subsequently became aware of the faux pas I had made. I became canny of an important aspect of what it means to make a good life in Spey Bay. Although I have certainly bought ethically questionable food items since returning from fieldwork, I still carry out ethical audits when I am shopping now; once learned, the habit is hard to shake off.

People in Spey Bay try to shop ethically, though they also acknowledge that choosing items requires knowledge and careful consideration of the complex structures of contemporary food markets and often a commitment to spending more. There is a sense of shared purpose, though, in the striving. Through ethical labour, people in Spey Bay make community—a community of like-minded, or similarly ethical, people. They try to make a better future. The work of the wildlife centre does not make anything in terms of a product or object, but it is highly productive. Like ethical shopping, it produces a sense of shared responsibility, it articulates ethical imperatives, and it shapes visions of a good future. For the staff, it makes ethical and professional identities and it helps make life good. Volunteers give their time to the wildlife centre because they want to do something good and because volunteering is a way of enacting the positive attributes that are commonly associated with rural living—building belonging, forging bonds with other people, caring for the environment.[29] They create value through their time and ethical labour, and by doing so together, and in consultation with each other, they make community.

In her study of artisanal cheese-makers in the United States, Heather Paxson has described how economic, ethical, and social logics inform and are intertwined with each other in the making and selling of cheese. She argues that, for these small-scale cheese-makers, their attempts to realise and reconcile competing ethics are themselves a source of value. As she puts it, "It is the moral struggle, and not necessarily its resolution, that makes artisanship worth undertaking."[30] Artisanal cheese is a product that is bought and sold, but although its makers often struggle to make a living, its production and exchange are not solely guided by the logics of capitalism. But, like people in Spey Bay, artisan cheese-makers are not moral purists either. They are driven to cheese-making and dairy farming in order to get away from some elements of contemporary capitalist urban life, yet they are not practising Thoreauvian experiments in going back to the land. They have brought derelict farms back into production and enjoy living and working "closer to nature," but they do not necessarily reject industrial machinery, espouse organic principles, or balk at commodifying their story for marketing purposes.

Along with an increasing amount of attention to ethics in recent scholarship there have also been a number of attempts to capture the contingency of everyday life and ethical decision making. In her previous work on motherhood in urban Greece, Paxson described being a good woman as a system of virtues.[31] Around the same time, Charis Thompson applied the concept of choreography to the ways in which Americans approach participating in fertility treatment, which she has extended in her recent work on stem cell research.[32] Before that, Rayna Rapp described women undergoing amniocentesis as moral pioneers.[33] Annemarie Mol has led the charge in describing care and acts of caring as tinkering.[34] Most recently, Cheryl Mattingly has developed the concept of moral laboratories to capture the experimentation at the heart of ethics and family life.[35] All of these ways of articulating what I have referred to as the contingency of ethics are helpful, and the fact that different theorists use different terms for their particular contexts is in keeping with the point that ethics are neither static nor universal. What each of these terms expresses is a sense of movement and change, and by placing my emphasis on *making*—making ethics, making ethical decisions, making a good life—I am similarly trying to get across the point that ethics is always being made and always a question of context, and that to understand ethics, we must understand how it is made. Like the cheese-makers Paxson describes, people in Spey Bay select amongst elements of the urban and rural, the commercial and the pastoral, the economic and the social, and in this way they make daily decisions about what is natural and what is ethical. They are cannily living out the balancing act of making a good life.

// You've Been Trumped!

At the start of the twentieth century, the golf resort was the most important industry in Spey Bay alongside the salmon fishing at Tugnet. The golf links and hotel were originally built in 1907 and this was by all accounts a popular leisure destination, with the Lossiemouth-born former British prime minister Ramsay MacDonald a regular player in the 1920s, so there has in fact been over a century of tourism in the village. However, this declined during World War II, when the hotel was requisitioned for RAF troops based at Nether Dallachy, one mile southeast of Spey Bay. The hotel was largely destroyed in a fire in 1965 and later rebuilt with little of its former grandeur.[1]

In the film *Local Hero* (Forsyth, 1983), which was filmed in Pennan, on the Moray Firth coast, a Texas oil company attempts to buy the village and its coastline to develop a refinery. I was reminded of the film, which is a favourite of mine, when I first heard about the plans of American entrepreneur and political dabbler Donald Trump to develop a golf and leisure complex near Balmedie on the Aberdeenshire coast,[2] which have been resisted by local environmental groups including the charity in Spey Bay.[3] Their objections are based on the project's siting on environmentally sensitive land, part of which is a Site of Special Scientific Interest. Trump, who was keen to emphasise his family roots in Scotland throughout the process,[4] planned to spend £1 billion on a golf resort that he claimed would be "the greatest in the world." No one doubted that this could bring considerable amounts of money to an area of Scotland that is in need of investment, though many local people were sceptical that the money would trickle down to ordinary people.

There was a feeling amongst people in Spey Bay that the Trump case was an example of local government being swayed from taking the ethical course of action, namely protecting the natural world from exploitation, by the lure of money. Whilst they did not suggest in so many words that those who agreed to the proposal were corrupt, they did see a clear link between "greed" and approval for the plans. When the plans had first been presented to the local council's infrastructure services committee in November 2007, they had been defeated by one member's vote against them. The people I knew in Spey Bay saw this man's action as a triumph for moral integrity and bravery, reflecting their awareness that financial incentives may be hard to resist for most people and that standing up for your principles can entail sacrifice; indeed he was sacked from the committee shortly after the vote.

For many local residents, Trump's claims to Scottishness rang somewhat hollow, and this is probably less to do with his criterion—the rather compelling fact of his mother's roots on the Isle of Lewis—than with what would be at stake in accepting it. Media coverage of the project was mixed, reflecting competing pressures to protect the environment and invest in rural areas. There was a suggestion in some quarters that locals directly affected by the development were motivated by parochialism, and there may be an added issue of class tension as Aberdeen is one of the most affluent cities in the UK yet there are also pockets of severe economic deprivation in the city and surrounding county. Golf, though a Scottish invention, is a rich man's sport, which Trump's luxury complex does little to dispel. People in Spey Bay, however, tended to focus on preventing the apparently inevitable damage the development would cause to an area of coastline that they described to me as unique, special, and rare. In backing their claims, they pointed to its SSSI status and the responsibility to protect the area that that entails, suggesting this was an obvious ethical, and legal, imperative. As such, their ire was focused not so much on Trump—they didn't expect him to care about the land, the environment, or other people—but on the apparently morally corrupt *local* government officials who were, it seemed to them, so quick to override environmental safeguards in pursuit of short-term economic benefit.

After the development's embattled course through the local council planning system, the Scottish Government stepped in in late 2007, claiming that, because of its importance and potential contribution to the Scottish economy, the development required national scrutiny. After some back and forth between ministers and councillors about the propriety with which the whole affair had been conducted, Trump International Golf Links Scotland was eventually opened in 2012. But plans to open a new hotel and second course on the site, for which they also received planning permission in 2012, have been on hold since it was announced that the Scottish Government was backing the development of an offshore wind farm in Aberdeen Bay, which Donald Trump said would spoil the view from the golf course.[5]

In 2012, the same year that Trump International Golf Links Scotland officially opened, Michael Forbes, a local resident who refused to move from his home in the middle of the planned development and who became the figurehead of opposition to it, won "Top Scot" in the Glenfiddich Spirit of Scotland Awards. Various newspapers reported that Donald Trump was livid at this decision and had accused William Grant & Sons of rigging the vote because they were worried about competition from Trump's recently launched own brand of Scotch whisky, which will be served in-house on the golf estate. After Glenfiddich refused to apologise for Forbes's award, which they pointed out was determined by a public vote, Trump banned any products made by William Grant & Sons from his entire hotel and leisure empire.[6] Commentators speculated that, as the largest Scotch producer in the world, Glenfiddich could probably afford to stand its ground.

6

A Stable Environment

Ordinary writing is an experiment
in what you know.

—*Sarah Franklin*

Ethicising Reproduction, Reproducing Ethics

In exploring what people in Spey Bay think about the ethics of
reproduction and ART in this book, my aim has been to parse
out what reproductive ethics is, not only in the sense of what
people judge to be good but also in terms of what counts as belonging to the domain of ethics. Why is it that reproduction and
ethics seem to be so strongly wedded to each other? The answers
to this question are in many ways obvious, but then, it is often
the most obvious answers that require social scientists' attention.
Reproduction is about creating new life. It is, for many, the most
natural thing in the world—the facts of life, the fulfilment of
biological destiny, the continuation of the species. One does not
have to look far to find these notions—they are the low-hanging
fruit of British ideas about having children. Rather than taking
these ideas as clichés, as an ethnographer I am compelled to take
them seriously, to try to get at what these rather abstract and
philosophical ideas mean.

Reproduction creates new lives in the form of children, certainly, but what it also does is provide an opportunity for people to express, and put into action, the values that they believe
make life good. This is why, for example, (potential) parents
who carry genes for horrendous rare diseases insist they are only
using pre-implantation genetic diagnosis to give their children

the "advantage" of living a normal life span without an unusual amount of ill health or discomfort,[1] whilst the spectre of parents selecting amongst in vitro embryos provokes agonised questions about "designer babies" and the limits of parental involvement in determining the makeup[2] of their children amongst the wider public. Reproduction can be seen as an ethical microcosm, as a model for how life should be, and whilst any one particular act of reproduction may be most significant for the resulting child and her parents, it has wider effects, too, because how we reproduce seems to say something about who we are and who we want to be and because of a sense that future generations are the product of parents' reproductive decision making.

Another common feature of public debates about ART is the idea that people who cannot reproduce through heterosexual intercourse should not jump straight to ART but also think about adoption, fostering, co-parenting, kinship care, or even embracing childlessness. Whilst there is much to be said for remembering that ART are not the only answer to childlessness, it is also patently unfair to put responsibility for the world's parentless children onto any specific group (and especially so when that group is already subject to stigma and unequal access to resources). Once again, this example reminds us that debates about reproduction are metonymic of debates about life more generally. Reproduction models ethical values and ethical labour. In Spey Bay, the key values people associated with "good" reproduction and parenthood were responsibility, care, and altruism and one way they expressed this was in the hope that people—and not necessarily only the infertile or single-sex couples—would consider adoption or fostering before turning to assisted conception.

Neither ethics nor reproduction fits within disciplinary bounds. Debates about ART flow between questions of personhood, identity, morality, science, genetics, economics, politics, law, time, nature, and more. Reproduction is profoundly boundless and the questions it raises are ubiquitous. This is also true of ethics. Thinking about ethics requires following connections, however promiscuous or unruly they might appear. Ethical conversations are often uncomfortable because they trouble usual boundaries of propriety, lead to unexpected places, and typically show no deference for disciplinary domaining.

Ethnography, Ethics, and Emotion

One of the best ways of getting at ethics, of following its fluid flow as it is made and reproduced, is talking. Data, in ethnographic fieldwork, are not latent in our interlocutors, waiting to be unearthed by the researcher; they come from the space between the ethnographer and participant.[3] To use an environmentalist metaphor, gathering data is not about extracting a commodity but responsibly harnessing a renewable resource by redirecting its flow. If data are to be found in the gaps between interlocutors, then we must carefully mind those gaps.

In this ethnography I have developed the concept of ethical labour to describe some of the characteristics of the everyday work that goes into making a good life in Spey Bay. I have focused to a larger extent on the ethical labour of people living in Spey Bay, but the chapters have been punctuated by reflections on my own ethnographic, emotional, and ethical labour whilst I was there. Ethics is profoundly emotional, and this is another reason why Hochschild's work on emotional labour is significant to what I am describing here. The public ethics of ART has commonly centred on visceral reactions and often it is difficult for people to explain why something is unethical except to say that it simply *feels* wrong. At the same time, understanding why something might be ethical for someone else requires feeling empathy[4] for their take on the world. Ethnography and ethics both require feeling the way, trusting our instincts about what to say and do in a given context. Listening to feelings and recognising when we have transgressed feeling rules can be a way of mapping the ethical terrain. The ability to read feeling rules depends in large part on empathy and identification, and the authority in transcribing them depends on trust and legitimacy, which is made through emotional engagements.

Maternal bonding is an important part of the stories we tell about reproduction, parenting, and kinship. It is also, as I explored in chapters 3 and 4, a way of describing—and prescribing—the natural and the ethical. In *After Nature*, Strathern discusses the loving bond that should exist between parents and which is thought to properly drive the instinct to produce children,[5] as well as the downward flow of emotion that a mother is supposed to experience towards her child, which not only sets up a stable environment for the child's development but is also an expression of the child's individuality, which is, as Strathern points out, a tenet of British kinship.[6] As I suggested in chapter 4, emotions also provide clues to ethics—people in Spey Bay worried that a surrogate mother might change her mind about relinquishing the child she has borne because the feeling of maternal bonding had become too strong to resist, but they also worried about the emotional harm this might inflict on the intended parents who have invested their hopes of becoming parents in her body.

To the field, I brought not only my training in social anthropology and native knowledge of Scottish and British culture but also my own ethical values, general knowledge, and emotional capacities. These all influenced the questions I asked, the relationships I made, the sympathy I elicited, and the empathy I offered. In the British cultural imagination, reproduction, parenthood, kinship, and emotion are quintessentially feminine. I must admit that it has therefore been tempting not to dwell too long on the importance of emotions in what people in Spey Bay said in my discussions with them, for fear of reproducing the sense that reproduction and emotions are all women's work and therefore that, by virtue of my own gender, they are naturally mine. Yet not addressing questions of emotion would be empirically negligent. My struggle with people in Spey Bay's biologically determinist ideas about child care and the way it added a sourness to my overarching sympathy with them is apparent in the discussion in chapter 3. But it seems to me that it would be unethical not to pay attention to what they said even if I do not agree with it, even if some self-righteous part of me wanted them to be "better" than that.

Sara Ahmed exhorts us to think not about what emotions are so much as what they *do* and suggests paying attention to how emotions circulate as well as where they "stick."[7] She also reminds us that "emotionality as a claim *about* a subject or a collective is clearly dependent on relations of power, which endow 'others' with meaning and value."[8] This point is demonstrated by my example here of people in Spey Bay talking with me about surrogacy and maternal bonding. Many of them did not have children at the time of those conversations and none of them had been involved in surrogacy arrangements, so they were attributing the emotions of maternal bonding to others as part of a speculative exercise. As I said in chapter 4, much of what they said about maternal bonding can be read as an expression of their ethical values as much as their apprehension of the realities of maternal bonding. And in describing their gendered ideas about parenting, I am performing another iteration of this; a difference in opinion and the disappointment it made me feel forced me to recognise them as other and that in itself is something of a loss.

Making Natural Connections

But to return to the question with which I started, what is it about reproduction that seems to provoke attention to the ethical? What does the bringing together of reproduction, nature, and ethics do and what does it tell us about each?

There is a danger, and an opportunity, with merographic connections of making the connections that people use to make sense of and express their view of the world appear "only" metaphorical. That is, with merographic connections, one domain may be connected with another in people's thoughts and speech, but that connection may also at any time be broken. Merographic connections are playful, experimental. Jenny talked about fish that have changed sex because of environmental pollutants in an answer to a question I asked her about contemporary determinants of human (in)fertility. Responding to the same question, Sophie demonstrated her knowledge about the superior breeding efficiency of farm animals to suggest that humans may one day become an endangered species. Both of these answers could be read as horribly bleak, as pointing forward to human extinction brought about by irresponsibility and poor planning. Or they could be read as somewhat melodramatic metaphors, a way of warning about what might, but which has not yet and may never, happen. They could, indeed, be read as a way of sidestepping my question, of making clear what they think are the important issues facing the world, whatever I might have been trying to get at in my deliberately vague question. There are plenty of other possible readings, too. One responsibility I have as an ethnographer is in getting across the ambivalence that is at the heart of people's responses to ART, and one way I have tried to do that is by letting people speak for themselves as much as possible through the connections they make. Being a good ethnographer is about asking good questions, but to find the "right" questions, we have to listen to the answers. Perhaps this is why the findings of ethnographic research are often, simply, better questions.[9]

In the introduction, I noted the feature of merographic connections that Franklin calls "analogic return," which conveys the sense that in knowledge as in anything else, reproduction always contains an element of individuality or diversity. Similarly, in *Reproducing the Future*, Strathern writes:

> In cultural life, in those habits of thought about which for most of the time we are very much unaware, the ideas that reproduce themselves in our communications *never reproduce themselves exactly*. They are always found in environments or contexts that have their own properties or characteristics. These environments or contexts provide a range of domains.

We can think of all the social differences that opportunity, class, gender, expertise and so forth make to how the world is perceived; interests such as these form several such environments, and profoundly shape the nature of communication. Moreover, insofar as each is a domain, each imposes its own logic of "natural" association. Natural association *means* that ideas are always enunciated in an environment of other ideas, in contexts already occupied by other thoughts and images. Finding a place for new thoughts becomes an act of displacement.[10]

In associating gender-bending fish with infertile humans, Jenny hoped to express—amongst other things—her knowledge about the interconnectedness of humans, non-human animals, and the environment. But what happens to the fish that are used in this example when they are made to stand for something else, whether future human endangerment, changing genders and biologies, or the unfettered flow of water around the globe? Once associated with other environments or contexts, some of those associations stick. The sense that we live in an interconnected environment becomes real, as do the stickier associations—the ones that seem natural.

There is also an ethical, and political, element to such associations. In order to be known, something must first be recognised and domains must be apprehended as having their own contexts in order to be brought into relation. It is because of these different contexts that merographic connections can be made at all—connection relies on differentiation as much as association. Merographic connections make knowledge by pushing through boundaries, by flowing like water across domains. Each new merographic connection ripples out into the domains that are brought together and this is important, as Strathern points out, because culture, which is made through such connections, "has its constraints and effects on how people act, react and conceptualise what is going on around them," as "it is the way people imagine things really are."[11]

In this book, I have used ethnography to show the broad reach of ideas about reproduction and to illustrate its centrality to human life. I have worked from the premise that although the many studies of the experience of infertility and its medical treatment amongst patients and practitioners of the last three decades have huge empirical and theoretical value, there is still a dearth of information about what reproduction and ART mean for people who do not have personal experience of using these technologies. Their perspectives are important because public conversations about reproductive ethics have been dominated by interested parties and by crude adversarial arguments. They are significant not only because ART are a platform for further biotechnological and medical innovations but also because they have the capacity to effect deep social, cultural, ethical, biological, and ontological changes, though not in the simplistic ways that either doomsday or progressivist accounts might have us believe. The question of the ethics of ART is not whether people should be allowed to access medical treatments for infertility, which is a facile and by this point redundant one, but what the broader effects of such interventions into "life itself" are, whether that be for conjugal relations, parenting culture, gendered experiences of work, kinship, genetics, biology, industry, the environment, or the future of humanity.

My point is not to dismiss people who are using ART as biased, nor is it to imply that people who have not had that specific experience are more objective. It is instead to show that we all work within certain contexts and it is the ethnographer's job to elucidate these contexts. It should, then, be clear that I am not claiming that this book offers an exemplary way of studying reproduction or a model context in which to understand reproduction. If anything, I am suggesting that because reproduction reaches across domains, it can in fact be found everywhere and studied anywhere.

Jeanette Edwards has written about returning to Bacup to talk with people about ART and genetic technologies a decade after her original research for *Born and Bred*, her study of Lancashire kinship and attitudes to ART. She reflects that many of the ways in which people in Bacup talked about these technologies rested on similar premises as they had in their previous conversations. As she says, these perennial issues of identity, kinship, class, trust in experts, and so on remain salient because "they are prisms through which innovative and novel technologies are apprehended and transformed into objects of knowledge, which then cast a different light on the intricacies of social relationships."[12] Edwards seeks to problematise the "deficit" model of public understanding of science and genetics in particular. She says:

> There is clearly a need for more effective ways of hearing what people are saying about genetics: for taking what they say seriously. This means taking seriously those things which at first glance do not look like science. If we always treat scientific knowledge as a different order from, say, the knowledge required to sustain and maintain appropriate relationships between persons (and places and things), then we will continue to ignore the connections people make, which at the very least belie their ignorance.[13]

As Edwards suggests, the public understanding of science need not be a one-way flow of information from experts to laypeople. Perhaps instead each could take the other seriously.

Future Regenerations

The context for this study of reproduction and ART is one of everyday concern for the present and future state of the natural world. I did not go to northeast Scotland looking for environmentalists, but people's ideas about the environment proved a fruitful context in which to reflect on the ways in which reproduction reaches across domains. In assessing reproductive ethics, people in Spey Bay drew on the same sorts of values that guided their everyday lives: responsibility, community, stability, care, naturalness. Reproduction and environmentalism are both future oriented, and in thinking about each, people in Spey Bay considered what effects present actions might have on future generations. Reproduction and environmentalism are both concerned with life and oriented towards making good lives. As we saw in chapter 2, people's concerns about the potential long-term consequences of technological assistance to human reproduction point to an endangered future in which the expected link between generativity and futurity could become denatured. In this scenario, the common idea that children are their parents' future would become a negative, destructive, and potentially even apocalyptic relationship. As the spectre of species endangerment makes clear, the inability to reproduce is tragic because it is an ultimate ending since the hope that future generations represent is erased completely.

In his history of environmentalism, Joachim Radkau has noted that environmentalism is characterised, within the contemporary "risk society," by a focus on hypothetical risks.[14] People in Spey Bay did not dwell on apocalyptic visions of the future or delight in depicting doomsday scenarios, and their fears about the future of human reproduction were subtle and suggestive rather than certain or expectant. They did not assume that ART would lead to human endangerment but instead hoped that those with the power to do so considered such hypothetical risks when developing, promoting, and providing these treatments to infertile people.

People in Spey Bay were not extreme in their adherence to environmental ethics, much as they worried about the future of the planet. Their everyday ethics reflect a striving for stability, and this is true of their attitudes towards technology as much as anything. Their fears that humans are creating a potentially bleak future for ourselves by attempting to control our reproduction through technology reflect concerns about runaway scientific "progress" and the limits of biology, but they also point to ambivalence about choice and human nature. This ambivalence is represented in their everyday lives and work by the plight of whales and dolphins, which not only are victims of human activity but also act as ethical containers for the kinds of values and behaviours that they would like to pass on to their own and future generations.

In articulating their reproductive ethics, people in Spey Bay were also delineating their ideas about the limits of nature and the responsibilities that people have towards protecting it. They were comfortable expressing their ideas about reproduction through the idiom of naturalness and referred to nature as a grounding concept in articulating their ethics. But ART also exposes the fact that natural forces may come into conflict with each other, as in the biological urge to have children versus the danger of using technology that may ultimately reproduce infertility or prevent children in need from being adopted. In considering a future in which people have become overreliant on technology to reproduce, people in Spey Bay worried that there would be a cumulative effect of choices that favour individual wants over collective goods, or human desires over natural needs. For them, choices are never isolated from contexts and the future is the cumulative effect of those choices, which can build up like waste or pollution and create unforeseen consequences.

//

Tim Ingold has recently launched a provocative broadside against the "overuse" of the term "ethnography" in academia.[15] In making this critique, he draws a distinction between participant observation and ethnography:

> To practice participant observation . . . is to join in correspondence with those with whom we learn or among whom we study, in a movement that goes forward rather than back in time. Herein lies the educational purpose, dynamic, and potential of anthropology. As such, it is the very opposite of ethnography, the descriptive or documentary aims of which

impose their own finalities on these trajectories of learning, converting them into data-gathering exercises destined
to yield "results," usually in the form of research papers or
monographs.[16]

Ingold's argument is charmingly curmudgeonly. As ever, he
puts across his point in a highly engaging way, and given my
own sense of the importance of context, I do have sympathy
with his reservations about scholars—and, for that matter,
market researchers—blithely coupling "ethnography" with
other terms, as in "ethnographic interviews" and "ethnographic
theory," gratifying as it is to see ethnographic research methods
having their day in the sun. But I would not draw such a sharp
distinction between participant observation and ethnography.
There is, certainly, a difference in what is made by participant
observation and what is made by ethnography, but I wonder
how meaningful that difference is given their interconnected
nature. After all, each is usually made by the same person. Participant observation and ethnographic writing are, whilst qual-
itatively different activities, necessarily entangled in each other.

I would be surprised if many anthropologists manage to
keep ethnography out of their thoughts whilst practicing participant observation. It would be impossible—in Ingold's view of
ethnography, as my own—to become an ethnographer without
doing participant observation. Participant observation makes
"data," but it also makes a participant observer, who makes an
ethnography. Ethnography and ethnographer are both products of participant observation. As someone who did participant observation amongst people with similar socioeconomic
positions to me, fieldwork felt like correspondence, so Ingold's
use of this term to describe participant observation rings true
to my experience in Spey Bay. But the process of writing this
ethnography myself makes me wonder how feasible—not
to mention helpful or accurate—it is to distinguish between
when one is an anthropologist or sociologist and when one is
an ethnographer.

In many ways it feels like I have been in correspondence with the people I knew in Spey Bay as I have written here what they told me, what I observed of their lives, how I came, temporarily, to make a good life of my own in Spey Bay alongside them and with their guidance. This is not to deny that, in writing this down and publishing it, I have the authority as author, that I am the one who gets to tell people what life in Spey Bay was like, whilst I was there. But acknowledging that privilege also does not undo the fact that, in making this ethnography, I have endeavoured to get across the constant striving for the good that was a part of life there. And that striving is, as I have said, future oriented. The project of making a good life is a constant process, and it only takes a little imagination to see that an ethnography can be both finished and unfinished, too. It is one conversation in a relationship, one or two years out of a life, one dish eaten at a feast. When we look at a photograph, we do not think that the life or landscape it captures is final, that it has ended with its documentation; there is no reason why we should think that about ethnography either. Life has continued in Spey Bay— people have come and gone, babies have been born and children have grown up, the dolphins still feed at the mouth of the Spey and some part of me will always belong there. The river flows towards the sea; the sea swells and falls on the shore.

NOTES

Prologue

1. See http://www.gov.scot/Resource/Doc/1221/0052925.pdf.
2. Sperm whales do not use their teeth for eating, instead sucking squid and other prey straight into their mouths. Scientists often use the teeth to measure the age of beached whales as they form rings that indicate the number of years a whale has been alive, much like a tree. Whalers, meanwhile, favoured sperm whales' teeth for scrimshaw work.
3. Parsons 2012.
4. Spermaceti was used for lighting, as a lubricant, and as an excipient in pharmaceuticals and cosmetics. It is no longer available given the international moratorium on commercial whaling, but at a talk given by Philip Hoare in 2014, I learned that spermaceti is still used as a lubricant in NASA's telescopes and spaceships because of its low freezing point.
5. Beale 1839.
6. Hoare 2008: 75.
7. Ibid., 74–75.
8. Ibid., 78.

Introduction

1. Edwards 2002.
2. Bell 2014.
3. Franklin 2013: 61.
4. See Franklin 1997, 2013.
5. See Spallone and Steinberg 1987; Stanworth 1991; Pfeffer 1993.
6. See Cooper and Waldby 2014 for more on translation, fertility treatments, and regenerative medicine.
7. Williams 2004 [1974].
8. Ibid., 133.
9. Cooper and Waldby 2014: 14.
10. See also Wilson 2011a, 2011b, 2014.
11. Kleinman 1999: 70.
12. Ibid., 71.
13. Callahan 1999.
14. See Das 1999.

15. Hoffmaster 2001.

16. Ibid., 2.

17. Ibid.

18. Wilson 2013.

19. Wilson 2011a: 123.

20. Wilson 2014; see also Strathern 1992a on individualised morality in Thatcherite Britain.

21. Wilson 2014.

22. Thompson 2005: 209–10. See also Williams 2004 [1974]: 49–50 on the limitations of the British media when it comes to representing "public opinion."

23. Thompson 2005: 210–11.

24. For more examples of ethnographies that take this kind of approach to ethics, reproduction, and kinship, see Mattingly 2014; Paxson 2004; Ginsburg 1989.

25. Mol, Moser, and Pols 2010: 13.

26. See Gilligan 1982, especially for how this relates to gender.

27. Many species of cetacean are endangered and the Yangtze River dolphin is thought to have become extinct in the last decade. But bottlenose dolphins are not, in fact, endangered and seem to have a relatively stable global population (IUCN 2012). They are, however, a protected species under the EU's Habitats Directive and Appendix II of the Convention on the International Trade in Endangered Species of Wildlife Flora and Fauna (CITES), as they represent "species that are not necessarily now threatened with extinction but that may become so unless trade is closely controlled" (CITES n.d.). Though they may not be currently endangered, bottlenose dolphins in Spey Bay stand as compelling mnemonics of people's fears about the irrevocable damage human activities wreak on the planet.

28. See "Moray Firth Special Area of Conservation," Moray Firth Partnership, http://www.morayfirth-partnership.org/sac.html.

29. Williams 1975; Strathern 1992a.

30. *Laich* is Scots for low-lying land.

31. The BBC documentary series *Trawlermen* also gives a fascinating insight into the lives and work of those in the contemporary fishing industry in Peterhead and Fraserburgh, at the southeastern edge of the Moray Firth. It did, however, attract some controversy because of the decision by the producers to provide subtitles for some of the men, who had particularly strong accents that might be difficult to follow against a backdrop of noisy machinery and stormy waves. See "Subtitle Decision 'Puzzles' Scots," BBC News Online, 4 August 2006.

32. Nadel-Klein 2003.

33. Davies et al. 2010.

34. Scott and Parsons 2005; Howard and Parsons 2006.

35. See Radkau 2014 for some informative and comprehensive timelines of the environmental movement and the influence of environmentalism and conservationism on international politics and culture.

36. Cassidy 2002.

37. Parsons 2012.

38. Ibid.

39. I have changed people's names in the interests of anonymity.

40. The Crown Estate is the property management company instituted by an Act of Parliament that deals with assets and land legally owned by the Sovereign.

41. Veg-boxes have become popular in the UK in the last few years; they can revitalise business for small-scale farmers and provide for consumers of a more "ethical" bent. A local farmer delivers the boxes in Spey Bay fortnightly. The fruit and vegetables are all certified organic and mostly seasonal produce from his farm, though he also offers sidelines like organic chocolate, meat, and dairy products.

42. See also Strathern 1992a: 22, 30.

43. Differences in types of job and volunteer position are explained further in chapter 1.

44. Scotland's Census—Area Profiles, http://www.scotlandscensus.gov .uk/ods-web/area.html.

45. Taylor 2008. This pattern has created tensions between native residents and incomers in some areas, with the common perception that counterurban migration to rural areas drives up housing prices, effectively preventing longstanding residents and their children from getting a foothold on the "property ladder." Such feelings were largely absent in Moray—perhaps partly because house prices are still very low compared to those in many other parts of the UK and rural Scotland has quite a sparse population but also, I would suggest, because of the area's long history of migration.

46. Watson 2003: 80.

47. Ibid., 71.

48. Ibid., 72.

49. Spey Bay *is* a very safe place, but this sense of safety was almost wilful at times, as when Sophie insisted on never locking her front door even after the wildlife centre was burgled one night in 2006.

50. Edwards 2000.

51. Cf. Nadel-Klein 2003.

52. Cf. Basu 2007; Macdonald 1997.

53. At this time, before the global financial crisis, British house prices were rising rapidly, especially in affluent and "up-and-coming" areas in

southeastern England and in and around the main cities. The first time I nosily inspected a local estate agent's window in late 2005, I saw that two-bedroom houses could be bought in Moray and Aberdeenshire for £80,000. I was shocked, and then a little tempted.

54. See Watson 2003: 77.

55. Indeed, as James Laidlaw (2014: 74) has pointed out, in Aristotelian ethics, "acting virtuously is not a means towards a distinct end of living a happy life. Acting virtuously constitutes a happy life."

56. Weston 1998: 76.

57. Ibid., 80.

58. See Cassidy 2002; Edwards 2000; Edwards and Strathern 2000.

59. See Carsten 2000.

60. Basu 2007.

61. See also Grove-White 1993.

62. In the UK, one of the reasons why people were particularly concerned about food production and provenance in the late twentieth and early twenty-first centuries is the experience of various national food crises that brought attention to worrisome aspects of industrial farming, including salmonella in eggs, bovine spongiform encephalopathy (BSE), and foot and mouth disease.

63. In the UK, perhaps the best-known sources of information on the ethical living movement are the writings of journalists Lucy Siegle and Leo Hickman, who have both been writing about these issues in the national newspaper *The Guardian* and in their own books for over a decade.

64. Recycling waste in Spey Bay encapsulates the fact that, whilst living somewhere so close to the natural world seems to lend itself to environmentalist action, it can also make it more difficult. Whereas in the London borough of Hackney, where I lived after returning from fieldwork, for example, the council provided recycling boxes to every household and took on the labour of sorting the waste themselves, in Spey Bay at the time of my fieldwork, we had to drive the waste for recycling two miles to the local tip, which had the nearest recycling facilities. People would often worry that the carbon emissions from these car journeys invalidated the act of recycling, but it was also tacitly recognised that a conservation charity could not stand by whilst its staff put all their waste into landfills and so we continued to take the recycling to the tip by car. In fact, taking on responsibility for removing the recycling for Sophie and the residential volunteers, which they were often reluctant to do themselves and which was easier for me because I had my own car, was one way in which I could do people a favour—and thereby ingratiate myself with them in the cause of my fieldwork.

65. Puig de la Bellacasa 2010.

66. Ibid., 157.

67. Puig de la Bellacasa 2012; see also Van Dooren 2014; Mol, Moser, and Pols 2010.

68. The steady rise in popularity of the Green Party in English and Scottish politics also rather gives the lie to the idea that environmentalism has become depoliticised in the shift towards ethical living.

69. Strathern 1992a: 197.

70. In thinking about environmentalism in Spey Bay, I have also found work in religious studies, including Rebecca Kneale Gould's (2005) study of homesteading and Sarah Pike's (2001) work on neo-pagans, both in the United States, useful. Not least, the contrasts with those movements and the people who live and work in Spey Bay have been a constant reminder of the small but fundamental differences in how people who might have similar values nonetheless conceive of nature and their relationship to the natural world in very different ways.

71. One interesting response to this challenge is Tim Choy's ethnography of environmentalism and endangerment in Hong Kong, *Ecologies of Comparison* (2011), which gives a lyrical sense of the ways in which the environment and environmental ideas permeate all aspects of life.

72. Milton 1993: 2–3; see also Berglund 1998.

73. O'Riordan 1981: ix, quoted in Milton 1993: 1.

74. Strathern 1992a.

75. Franklin 2013: 158.

76. Thompson 2005: 8.

77. http://www.oxforddictionaries.com/definition/english/context; emphasis added.

78. Strathern 1992a: 73.

79. Ibid., 8.

80. Van Dooren 2014: 293.

81. Franklin 2001, 2007.

82. Franklin 2014a.

83. See also Franklin 2013: 8.

Where the River Meets the Sea

1. Ingold 2000. See also Descola 2013; Hastrup 2013.

2. See also Strathern 1992a.

3. Ingold 2000: 50.

4. See, for example, Franklin et al. 2000.

5. See Haraway 2008.

Chapter 1

1. The term *ken* is characteristic of northeastern Scottish dialect and older people who have been resident in the area for a long time tend to pepper their speech with it. It literally means "know," and when used in conjunction with "you" or "ye" means "you know," although the "you" is often dropped, as it was here.

2. SeaWorld is a collection of three marine parks that exhibit dolphins and whales to the public in the United States.

3. Scottish Government 2010.

4. Ibid.

5. Franklin 1997; Ginsburg 1989; Paxson 2004; Rapp 1999.

6. Ginsburg and Rapp 1991: 322.

7. See also Paxson 2004.

8. Becker 1994: 391.

9. See Franklin 1997; Layne 1996; Strathern 1992a.

10. See also Mol, Moser, and Pols 2010.

11. Cooper and Waldby 2014; Mol, Moser, and Pols 2010.

12. Hochschild 2003: 7.

13. Ibid., 190.

14. Cooper and Waldby 2014.

15. Puig de la Bellacasa 2012; Van Dooren 2014.

16. Strathern 1988: 142, 152.

17. Day 2007.

18. Haraway 1991: 166.

19. Morini 2007.

20. Power 2009.

21. See Illouz 2007 for some parallels on Internet dating.

22. The parallels with the professional life of academics are probably too obvious to be worth mentioning, but they were especially apparent to me whilst I was carrying out fieldwork, where I felt I had to present myself as the open, empathetic, nonjudgemental participant observer at all times. Still, it felt worth it to me because I wanted to do good research and to pass my PhD. At the same time, I also felt guilty a lot of the time because spending my time hanging out with people often felt like it was a long way from being hard work.

23. See also Paxson 2004.

24. Hochschild 2003: 194.

Beginnings

1. More than one person has jokingly suggested to me that she was acting as a surrogate mother.

Chapter 2

1. See also Becker 1994; Franklin 1997; Layne 1996.

2. See Strathern 1992a: 39.

3. Choy 2011: 26–27.

4. Edwards 2000.

5. Scottish Government 2010.

6. Ibid.

7. See "NHS IVF Services to Be Fairer and Faster," Scottish Government, 15 May 2013, http://www.scotland.gov.uk/News/Releases/2013/05/IVF services15052013.

8. Scottish Government 2007.

9. Barnhart and Schreiber 2009.

10. Victoria Boydell (2010) carried out research amongst women in London who were using the oral contraceptive pill and found that the Pill enabled women to achieve some of the aspirations of contemporary femininity in terms of being good (future) mothers, workers, and lovers. But rather than simply freeing them up from their gender as some early champions of the Pill predicted, the technology also reentrenches ideas about the necessity of managing the "unruly" female body so that women can meet the demands of their multiple, gendered roles in the professional, domestic, familial, and conjugal spheres.

11. See, for example, National Institute of Environmental Health Sciences 2010.

12. Moore et al. 2011.

13. See di Chiro 2010; Scott 2009; Lamoreaux 2013.

14. Roberts 2007: 165.

15. Franklin 2013: 300–305.

16. Ibid., 301.

17. Ibid., 302.

18. Strathern 1992a.

19. Franklin 2013: 300.

20. Joanna, like some others, brought up the idea of "designer babies" in response to a rather broad question I had asked her about whether there were any examples of ART that she found unacceptable, and it should be clear that she was referring to the idea of parents selecting the genetic characteristics of their children for "social" reasons rather than using pre-implantation genetic diagnosis to prevent passing on a genetic disorder.

21. Laidlaw 2014; see also Faubion 2011.

22. See Foucault 1997.

23. Lambek 2010.

24. Laidlaw 2002: 317.

25. Robbins 2012: para. 18.
26. Macnaghten and Urry 1998: 143, 147.
27. Ibid., 152.
28. Franklin 2014b: 117.
29. Ibid., 113.
30. Strathern 1992a; see also Strathern 1992b: 28.
31. Strathern 1992a: 195.
32. Franklin 2013, 2003.
33. Williams 1977.

The Water of Life

1. Scotch Whisky Association 2011.
2. See Trubeck 2009.
3. "William Grant & Sons Breaks £1bn Turnover Barrier Again," *The Herald*, 30 September 2013.
4. Glenfiddich website, accessed 21 February 2014.
5. See Momus 2009 for a creative take on the idea of parallel Scottish worlds.

Chapter 3

1. Severin Carrell, "Free Marvin: Can Scaffolding and Fish Bait Save the Whale?" *The Guardian*, 3 August 2007.
2. See "Minke Whale Escapes from Harbor," BBC News Online, 3 August 2007. The story was also covered by *The Guardian*, *The Times*, and Channel Five news, amongst others.
3. See Cassidy 2002; Haraway 2008.
4. Throughout, I will use the term "maternal bonding" rather than "mother-child bond" to reflect the fact that in our discussions about parenthood and parenting, people in Spey Bay focused almost exclusively on the mother's relationship to her child rather than the child's relationship to her mother.
5. Erin and Duncan are unusual amongst the people I met in Spey Bay, as Catholics and as people who regularly attend church. The only other person who definitely defined herself as a Christian was Willow, though she did not regularly attend church in Moray because she found the way in which services were conducted did not fit with the small evangelical church she had joined as a teenager. Many others described themselves as agnostic, which in practice meant that they did not usually attend church but did not rule out religious ideas or belief in god. A handful of people were atheists.

6. Debendox is the UK brand name for Bendectin (Merrell Dow [no relation]), which was withdrawn from the U.S. market in 1983 after a series of lawsuits but has now been relaunched there as Diclegis (Duchesnay), which is approved by the FDA. Diclegis has the same constitution as Bendectin, an equal combination of doxylamine succinate and pyridoxine hydrochloride and is used to treat nausea and vomiting in pregnancy. A recent article in the *New England Journal of Medicine* states that the decision to withdraw the drug was "not science-based" (Slaughter et al. 2014: 1081) and suggests that the contemporary allegations that the drug was teratogenic were influenced by the recent thalidomide scandal, which fanned the flames of public concern. The authors write, "Courtroom testimony claiming that Bendectin was a human teratogen was markedly devoid of evidence-based corroboration. Merrell Dow indicated that its decision to withdraw Bendectin was based not on safety issues but on financial concerns. In the wake of the Bendectin allegations, the company's insurance premiums had risen to $10 million per year, only $3 million less than the total income from Bendectin sales" (2014: 1082).

7. See, in particular, Davis-Floyd 2004; Martin 2001; Oakley 1986.

8. See Lee et al. 2014.

9. See Hays 1996; Faircloth et al. 2013; Lee et al. 2014.

10. See Davis 2008; Eyer 1992; Faircloth 2013; Lee et al. 2014; Suizzo 2004; Taylor 1998; Wall 2001.

11. See Lee et al. 2014.

12. Davis 2008.

13. See Collier and Yanagisako 1987; Franklin 1997, 2013; Ginsburg and Rapp 1995; Schneider 1984; Strathern 1980, 1988, 1992a, 1992b; Yanagisako and Delaney 2013.

14. Franklin 1997; Strathern 1992a.

Arrivals

1. Milton 1993.
2. Strathern 1992a.
3. Rapport 2010: 80.
4. See also Kleinman 1999.

Chapter 4

1. Highland Council 2006.
2. See also Stoett 1997.

3. Perhaps, for the sake of setting the scene better, I should note here that I am only 5' 3" (161 cm) tall; Sophie is above-average height for a woman. I am also four years younger than Sophie.

4. See Anderson 1990; Corea 1985; Stanworth 1987; Zipper and Sevenhuijsen 1987 for some early and influential examples and Cooper and Waldby 2014 for a more recent approach.

5. See Cook et al. 2003; Edwards et al. 1993; Strathern 1992a, 1992b, 2003.

6. See, for example, Pande 2009, 2010.

7. Konrad 2005; Ragoné 1994; Strathern 2003.

8. Franklin 2013.

9. Cotton and Winn 1985.

10. Cannell 1990: 674.

11. Of course, the word "bond" has a further, financially inflected meaning, which is worth bearing in mind given the contentious debate over commercial surrogacy.

12. Cf. Warnock 1985a: 47.

13. Drummond 1978: 40.

14. See also Strathern (2003, 1992b) for a discussion of whether the ethical dilemmas presented by surrogacy are as novel as they might at first appear.

15. See Ragoné 1994; Teman 2010; Thompson 2001.

16. Thompson 2005: 145.

17. Ibid., 177.

18. Susan Markens (2007) carried out a comparative study of surrogacy regulation in the states of New York and California. Of particular relevance to my analysis here is Markens's focus on "discursive frames" in the debates in each state. In both New York and California, both pro- and anti-surrogacy camps referred to "the best interests of the child" and the "freedom to choose" in making opposing arguments (see Edwards et al. 1993 for some parallels in the British debates around assisted conception in the 1980s and Ginsburg 1989 on the American abortion debate). Similarly, people in Spey Bay appealed to apparently stable concepts of genetics, biology, and nature but to make different and in some cases contradictory claims.

19. See Markens 2007; Satz 1992: 122; Stanworth 1987a: 27.

20. However, this is changing. At a recent talk, legal scholar Emily Jackson, who specialises in the regulation of ART, reported that British people are now turning to the Internet, online social networks, and foreign brokers to arrange surrogacy, which has led to an increase in the number of cases that end up in court because of invalid contracts, custody disputes, and uncertainty about the reach of laws across national borders.

21. See also Hirsch 1993.

22. Brinsden 2003.

23. Cannell 1990; see also Cotton and Winn 1985.

24. See Almeling 2011 for some parallel observations about egg and sperm donation in the United States.

25. Lutz 1988; see also Illouz 2007 on "emotional capitalism."

26. Lutz 1988: 4.

27. Hochschild 2003: 31.

28. Williams 1978.

29. Hochschild 2003.

30. Strathern 1992a: 138.

31. See Markens 2007; Edwards et al. 1999; Franklin 1997.

32. Mulkay 1997; see also Edwards et al. 2005.

33. Cohen 1989.

34. Strathern 1981.

35. See also Macdonald 1996; Rapport 1993; Edwards 2000; Cassidy 2002.

36. See also Basu 2007 on the "Scottish diaspora."

37. Strathern 2003: 290.

38. See Franklin 2013, 1993; Mulkay 1997.

39. Warnock 1985a.

40. The Surrogacy Arrangements Act 1985 covers all of the UK, but there is a slightly amended version of the section that defines the "meaning of 'surrogate mother', 'surrogacy arrangement' and other terms" that is different for Scotland. The difference is that in the definition of a surrogate mother, the intended parents' *rights* are emphasised in the Scottish version; their *responsibilities* as parents are emphasised in the equivalent place in the section covering England, Wales, and Northern Ireland. The sections covering provision and offences are the same, so it is fair to say that the law on surrogacy is essentially the same throughout the UK, except for the shorter length of time intended parents have to register the birth in Scotland.

41. Cf. Bonaccorso 2008 on Italy and Pande 2010 on India for two examples of what has happened in countries that have been slower to regulate ART.

42. COTS (Childlessness Overcome Through Surrogacy) website, http://www.surrogacy.org.uk/registering-birth.htm.

43. See Blyth and Potter 2003; Brazier et al. 1998.

44. Ragoné 1994: 59.

45. Ibid., 32; see also Healy 2006; Teman 2010; Almeling 2011.

46. Douglas 1990.

47. Mauss 1990.

48. Highers are the pre-university qualifications taken by tertiary education students in Scotland, the equivalent of English "A" levels.

49. Ragoné 1994: 124; see also Roberts 1998; Teman 2010.

50. Ragoné 1994: 124.

51. By "anonymous" she seems to mean not only a situation where the intended parents and surrogate mother remain completely unknown to each

other (in Ragoné's terms, a "closed" surrogacy arrangement) but also a commercial surrogacy arrangement where the intended parents and surrogate are unknown to each other prior to the agreement but become acquainted through surrogacy (an "open" surrogacy arrangement).

52. Konrad 2005.

53. Thompson 2001.

54. Warnock 1985b.

55. See, for example, Ginsburg 1989; Ragoné 1994; Ginsburg and Rapp 1995; Hays 1996; Rapp 1999; Paxson 2004; Lee et al. 2014.

Chapter 5

1. Edwards 2000: 33.

2. See also Almeling 2011; Barnes 2014.

3. Oxford English Dictionary online: http://www.oxforddictionaries.com/definition/english/canny.

4. That is, a surrogacy arrangement in which the surrogate mother is paid for her "service," which, as discussed in the previous chapter, is illegal in the UK but legal in some American states as well as a handful of European and Asian countries.

5. Parry and Bloch 1989; Strathern 1988.

6. Zelizer 1997.

7. Warnock 1985a: 46.

8. See also Wilkinson 2003.

9. These concerns about pricing up surrogates are pertinent, as ethnographies of gamete donation and surrogacy have shown. Although in the UK there is a flat fee for both eggs and sperm and surrogates can have only their expenses reimbursed, in many parts of the world, premiums are paid for gametes extracted from donors with desirable attributes such as high educational attainment, phenotypic characteristics that fit particular racial and/or aesthetic ideals, and an amenable or compliant attitude (see, for example, Almeling 2011; Cooper and Waldby 2014). As Cooper and Waldby suggest, this selection of traits, which may or may not in fact be heritable, reflects not only the degree of control and consumer choice present in the transnational infertility industry (which British people are increasingly participating in themselves) but also a wider move, also discussed in chapter 1, towards valuing an increasing range of personal qualities in employees that were deemed irrelevant in prior models of employment.

10. Kopytoff 1986: 83.

11. Ibid., 64.

12. Cooper and Waldby 2014.

13. Ibid., 5.

14. Wolfram 1989; see also Ragoné 1994: 51.

15. It was also reported at the time that the intended parents were American, when in fact they were Swedish.

16. Wolfram 1989.

17. This is despite the fact that there has been plenty of resistance to "baby-selling" in the United States, too, as well as the fact that commercial surrogacy is only legal in a handful of states. See Susan Markens's (2007) illuminating comparative study of surrogacy debate and regulatory process in California and New York.

18. Were I to go back and reinterview people in Spey Bay, I would be interested in asking them what they think about people donating tissues for stem cell research. At the time, I felt that asking them about blood donation was most appropriate as they were much more likely to have some personal experience of it, whilst stem cell research was still extremely new in public debates.

19. Titmuss 1997.

20. Ibid., 59.

21. Tutton 2002.

22. Ibid., 528.

23. Nicholas Whitfield (2013) has also written about blood donation in the UK with specific reference to Titmuss's work, showing how the ideology of the "pure gift" of blood donation came to the fore in World War II propaganda and was in fact not so much about the promotion of the pure gift as a response to encroaching commercialism but the result of "historical coincidence and mutual complicity" (2013: 96)—the creation of the figure of the anonymous recipient of blood came about as a response to changes in the blood transfusion system in which blood was now banked and stored and could be donated to multiple recipients rather than the earlier one-to-one donations. Through advertising campaigns that presented ideal types of recipient, including wounded soldiers and the victims of air raids, people could imagine what sort of person their donated blood might be helping without having to deal with a specific, known individual to whom they would have, according to the logic of the gift as described by Mauss, enduring ties. As Whitfield puts it, "Strategic anonymity was at the heart of interwar altruism" (2013: 98). The blood donation and transfusion system in mid-twentieth-century Britain thereby managed to strike the right balance between individual altruism and a generalised duty to the community or nation.

24. Carsten 2013.

25. Lambek 2008: 136.

26. See also Thompson 2002; Friese 2013.

27. Parry 1986: 468.

28. Ibid., 458.
29. See also Strathern 1981; Little 1997.
30. Paxson 2013: 8.
31. Paxson 2004: 11.
32. Thompson 2005, 2013.
33. Rapp 1999.
34. See Mol, Moser, and Pols 2010.
35. Mattingly 2014.

You've Been Trumped!

1. See Nalder 2000 for an enthusiastic description of playing golf at Spey Bay.

2. I was not the first person to see the parallel; see "Billionaire Donald Trump Faces Kilted Curmudgeon Opposing His Scottish Golf Resort Plans," *Daily Mail*, 21 October 2007.

3. Anthony Baxter also draws on this parallel in his revealing documentary about the affair, *You've Been Trumped* (2011).

4. See, in particular, "Donald Trump on Lewis: Aberdeen Golf Plan Is for My Mother," *The Herald*, 29 July 2008.

5. "Trump to Build New Club House Despite Wind Farm Row," *The Scotsman*, 7 August 2014.

6. See Severin Carrell, "Donald Trump's Scottish Love Affair on the Rocks after Whisky Award Slight," *The Guardian*, 5 December 2012.

Chapter 6

1. Franklin and Roberts 2006.
2. Edwards 2005.
3. Thanks to Juliet Rayment (2014) for articulating this point, which I paraphrase here from her paper given at De Montfort University on 5 December 2014.

4. See Carolyn Pedwell's recent (2014) book for an in-depth consideration of the politics of empathy.

5. Strathern 1992a: 156; see also Schneider 1968.
6. Strathern 1992a: 49, 125.
7. Ahmed 2013 [2004]: 4.
8. Ibid., 4, original emphasis.
9. Franklin and Roberts 2006.
10. Strathern 1992b: 6, original emphasis.

11. Ibid., 3.
12. Edwards 2002: 323.
13. Ibid., 324.
14. Radkau 2014: 149.
15. Ingold 2014: 383.
16. Ibid., 390.

BIBLIOGRAPHY

Ahmed, S. 2013 [2004]. *The Cultural Politics of Emotion*. Abingdon: Routledge.

Almeling, R. 2011. *Sex Cells: The Medical Market for Eggs and Sperm*. Berkeley: University of California Press.

Anderson, E. S. 2008. Is Women's Labor a Commodity? *Philosophy and Public Affairs* 19(1), 71–92.

Barnes, L. W. 2014. *Conceiving Masculinity: Male Infertility, Medicine, and Identity*. Philadelphia: Temple University Press.

Barnhart, K. T., and C. A. Schreiber. 2009. Return to Fertility Following Discontinuation of Oral Contraceptives. *Fertility and Sterility* 91(3), 659–63.

Basu, P. 2007. *Highland Homecomings: Genealogy and Heritage Tourism in the Scottish Diaspora*. Abingdon: Routledge.

Beale, T. 1839. *The Natural History of the Sperm Whale: To which is Added a Sketch of a South-Sea Whaling Voyage, in which the Author was Personally Engaged*. London: Manning and Mason.

Becker, G. 1994. Metaphors in Disrupted Lives: Infertility and Cultural Constructions of Continuity. *Medical Anthropology Quarterly* 8(4), 383–410.

Bell, A. V. 2014. Diagnostic Diversity: The Role of Social Class in Diagnostic Experiences of Infertility. *Sociology of Health & Illness* 36(4), 516–30.

Berglund, E. K. 1998. *Knowing Nature, Knowing Science: An Ethnography of Environmental Activism*. Cambridge: White Horse.

Billionaire Donald Trump Faces Kilted Curmudgeon Opposing His Scottish Golf Resort Plans. 2007. *Daily Mail Online*, 21 October. http://www.daily mail.co.uk/news/article-487384/Billionaire-Donald-Trump-faces-kilted -curmudgeon-opposing-Scottish-golf-resort-plans.html.

Blyth, E., and C. Potter. 2003. Paying for It? Surrogacy, Market Forces and Assisted Conception. In *Surrogate Motherhood: International Perspectives*, ed. R. Cook, S. D. Sclater, and F. Kaganas. Oxford: Hart Publishing.

Bonaccorso, M.M.E. 2009. *Conceiving Kinship: Assisted Conception, Procreation and Family in Southern Europe*. Oxford: Berghahn Books.

Boydell, V. 2010. The Social Life of the Pill: An Ethnography of the Oral Contraceptive Pill. Unpublished PhD thesis, London School of Economics.

Brazier, M., A. Campbell, and S. Golombok. 1998. *Surrogacy: Review for Health Ministers of Current Arrangements for Payments and Regulation—Report of the Review Team*. London: Department of Health. http://webarchive .nationalarchives.gov.uk/+/www.dh.gov.uk/en/Publicationsandstatistics /Publications/PublicationsLegislation/DH_4009697.

Brinsden, P. R. 2003. Clinical Aspects of IVF Surrogacy in Britain. In *Surrogate Motherhood: International Perspectives*, ed. R. Cook, S. D. Sclater, and F. Kaganas. Oxford: Hart Publishing.

Callahan, D. 1999. The Social Sciences and the Task of Bioethics. *Daedalus* 128(4), 275–94.

Cannell, F. 1990. Concepts of Parenthood: The Warnock Report, the Gillick Debate, and Modern Myths. *American Ethnologist* 17(4), 667–86.

Carrell, S. 2007. Free Marvin: Can Scaffolding and Fish Bait Save the Whale? *The Guardian*, 4 August. http://www.theguardian.com/uk/2007/aug/04 /topstories3.mainsection.

———. 2012. Donald Trump's Scottish Love Affair on the Rocks after Whisky Award Slight. *The Guardian*, 5 December. http://www.the guardian.com/world/2012/dec/05/donald-trump-whisky-award.

Carsten, J. 2000. "Knowing Where You've Come From": Ruptures and Continuities of Time and Kinship in Narratives of Adoption Reunions. *Journal of the Royal Anthropological Institute* 6(4), 687–703.

———. 2013. Introduction: Blood Will Out. *Journal of the Royal Anthropological Institute* 19:S1–S23. doi:10.1111/1467–9655.12013.

Cassidy, R. 2002. *The Sport of Kings: Kinship, Class and Thoroughbred Breeding in Newmarket*. Cambridge: Cambridge University Press.

Choy, T. 2011. *Ecologies of Comparison: An Ethnography of Endangerment in Hong Kong*. Durham, NC: Duke University Press.

CITES. The CITES Appendices. http://www.cites.org/eng/app/index.php.

Cohen, A. 1989. *Whalsay: Symbol, Segment and Boundary in a Shetland Island Community*. Manchester: Manchester University Press.

Collier, J. F. 1987. *Gender and Kinship: Essays toward a Unified Analysis*. Stanford: Stanford University Press.

Cook, R., S. D. Sclater, and F. Kaganas. 2003. *Surrogate Motherhood: International Perspectives*. Oxford: Hart Publishing.

Cooper, M., and C. Waldby. 2014. *Clinical Labor: Tissue Donors and Research Subjects in the Global Bioeconomy*. Durham, NC: Duke University Press.

Corea, G. 1985. *The Mother Machine: Reproductive Technologies from Artificial Insemination to Artificial Wombs*. New York: Harper and Row.

Cotton, K., and D. Winn. 1985. *Baby Cotton: For Love and Money*. London: Dorling Kindersley.

Council, H. 2006. *Residential and leisure development including housing, marina, boat yard, yacht club, visitors centre, nature conservation zones and hotel with supporting community facilities at Whiteness Head, Ardersier. Report by director of planning and development*. Inverness. www.highland.gov.uk /download/meetings/id/35895/item2reportpdf.

Das, V. 1999. Public Good, Ethics, and Everyday Life: Beyond the Boundaries of Bioethics. *Daedalus* 128(4), 99–133.

Davies, B., C. Pita, D. Lusseau, and C. Hunter. 2010. *The Value of Tourism Expenditure Related to the East of Scotland Bottlenose Dolphin Population: Final Report*. Aberdeen: Aberdeen Center for Environmental Sustainability.

Davis, K. 2008. "Here's Your Baby, on You Go": Kinship and Expert Advice amongst Mothers in Scotland. Unpublished PhD thesis, University of Edinburgh.

Davis-Floyd, R. E. 2004. *Birth as an American Rite of Passage: Second Edition, With a New Preface*. Berkeley: University of California Press.

Day, S. 2007. *On the Game: Women and Sex Work*. London: Pluto Press.

Descola, P. 2013. *Beyond Nature and Culture*. Chicago: University of Chicago Press.

Di Chiro, G. 2010. Polluted Politics? Confronting Toxic Discourse, Sex Panic, and Eco-Normativity. In *Queer Ecologies: Sex, Nature, Politics, Desire*, ed. C. Mortimer-Sandilands and B. Erickson, 199–230. Bloomington: Indiana University Press.

Donald Trump on Lewis: Aberdeen Golf Plan Is for My Mother. 2008. *The Herald*, 9 June. http://www.heraldscotland.com/donald-trump-on-lewis-aberdeen-golf-plan-is-for-my-mother-1.882182.

Douglas, M. 1990. Foreword: No Free Gifts. In *The Gift* by Marcel Mauss. London: Routledge.

Drummond, L. 1978. The Transatlantic Nanny: Notes on a Comparative Semiotics of the Family in English-Speaking Societies. *American Ethnologist* 5(1), 30–43.

Edwards, J. 2000. *Born and Bred: Idioms of Kinship and New Reproductive Technologies in England*. Oxford: Oxford University Press.

———. 2002. Taking "Public Understanding" Seriously. *New Genetics and Society* 21(3), 315–25.

———. 2005. "Make-up": Personhood through the Lens of Biotechnology. *Ethnos* 70(3), 413–31.

Edwards, J., and M. Strathern. 2000. Including Our Own. In *Cultures of Relatedness: New Approaches to the Study of Kinship*, 149–66. Cambridge: Cambridge University Press.

Edwards, J., S. Franklin, E. Hirsch, F. Price, and M. Strathern. 2005. *Technologies of Procreation: Kinship in the Age of Assisted Conception*. New York: Routledge.

Eyer, D. E. 1992. *Mother-Infant Bonding: A Scientific Fiction*. New Haven: Yale University Press.

Faircloth, C. 2013. *Militant Lactivism?: Attachment Parenting and Intensive Motherhood in the UK and France*. Oxford: Berghahn Books.

Faircloth, C., D. M. Hoffman, and L. L. Layne, eds. 2013. *Parenting in Global Perspective: Negotiating Ideologies of Kinship, Self and Politics*. Abingdon: Routledge.

Faubion, J. 2011. *An Anthropology of Ethics*. Cambridge: Cambridge University Press.

Foucault, M. 1997. *Ethics: Subjectivity and Truth*. London: Penguin Books.

Franklin, S. 1993. Postmodern Procreation: Representing Reproductive Practice. *Science as Culture* 3(4), 522–61.

———. 1997. *Embodied Progress: A Cultural Account of Assisted Conception*. Abingdon: Routledge.

———. 2001. Sheepwatching. *Anthropology Today* 17(3), 3–10.

———. 2002. *Embodied Progress: A Cultural Account of Assisted Conception*. London: Routledge.

———. 2003. Re-thinking Nature-Culture: Anthropology and the New Genetics. *Anthropological Theory* 3(1), 65–85.

———. 2007. *Dolly Mixtures: The Remaking of Genealogy*. Durham, NC: Duke University Press.

———. 2013. *Biological Relatives: IVF, Stem Cells, and the Future of Kinship*. Durham, NC: Duke University Press.

———. 2014a. Analogic Return: The Reproductive Life of Conceptuality. *Theory, Culture & Society* 31(2–3), 243–61.

———. 2014b. Rethinking Reproductive Politics in Time, and Time in UK Reproductive Politics: 1978–2008. *Journal of the Royal Anthropological Institute* 20(S1), 109–25.

Franklin, S., and C. Roberts. 2006. *Born and Made: An Ethnography of Preimplantation Genetic Diagnosis*. Princeton: Princeton University Press.

Franklin, S., C. Lury, and J. Stacey. 2000. *Global Nature, Global Culture*. London: Sage Publications.

Friese, C. 2013. *Cloning Wild Life: Zoos, Captivity, and the Future of Endangered Animals*. New York: New York University Press.

General Register Office for Scotland (GROS). 2010. *Grampian Migration Report*. http://www.nrscotland.gov.uk/files/statistics/migration/Migration-Reports/grampian-migration-report.pdf.

Gilligan, C. 1982. *In a Different Voice: Psychological Theory and Women's Development*. Cambridge, MA: Harvard University Press.

Ginsburg, F. D. 1989. *Contested Lives: The Abortion Debate in an American Community*. Berkeley: University of California Press.

Ginsburg, F. D., and R. Rapp, eds. 1995. *Conceiving the New World Order: The Global Politics of Reproduction*. Berkeley: University of California Press.

Gould, R. K. 2005. *At Home in Nature: Modern Homesteading and Spiritual Practice in America*. Berkeley: University of California Press.

Grove-White, R. 1993. Environmentalism: A New Moral Discourse for Technological Society? In *Environmentalism: The View from Anthropology*, ed. K. Milton, 18–30. London: Routledge.

Haraway, D. J. 1991. A Cyborg Manifesto: Science, Technology, and Socialist-Feminism in the Late Twentieth-Century. In *Simians, Cyborgs, and Women: The Reinvention of Nature*. London: Free Association Books.

———. 2008. *When Species Meet*. Minneapolis: University of Minnesota Press.

Hastrup, K., ed. 2013. *Anthropology and Nature*. Abingdon: Routledge.

Hays, S. 1996. *The Cultural Contradictions of Motherhood*. New Haven: Yale University Press.

Healy, K. 2010. *Last Best Gifts: Altruism and the Market for Human Blood and Organs*. Chicago: University of Chicago Press.

Hirsch, E. 1993. Negotiated Limits: Interviews in South-east England. In *Technologies of Procreation: Kinship in the Age of Assisted Conception*, ed. J. Edwards, S. Franklin, E. Hirsch, F. Price, and M. Strathern. London: Routledge.

Hoare, P. 2008. *Leviathan, or, The Whale*. London: Fourth Estate.

Hochschild, A. R. 2003. *The Managed Heart: Commercialization of Human Feeling, Twentieth Anniversary Edition, with a New Afterword*. Berkeley: University of California Press.

Hoffmaster, B. 2009. *Bioethics in Social Context*. Philadelphia: Temple University Press.

Howard, C., and E.C.M. Parsons. 2006. Attitudes of Scottish City Inhabitants to Cetacean Conservation. *Biodiversity and Conservation* 15(14), 4335–56.

Illouz, E. 2007. *Cold Intimacies: The Making of Emotional Capitalism*. Oxford: Wiley.

Ingold, T. 2000. *The Perception of the Environment: Essays on Livelihood, Dwelling and Skill*. London: Routledge.

———. 2014. That's Enough about Ethnography! *Hau: Journal of Ethnographic Theory* 4(1), 383–95.

IUCN. 2012. Tursiops truncatus. http://www.iucnredlist.org/details/22563/0.

Kleinman, A. 1999. Moral Experience and Ethical Reflection: Can Ethnography Reconcile Them? A Quandary for "The New Bioethics." *Daedalus* 128(4), 69–97.

Kleinman, A., R. C. Fox, and A. M. Brandt. 1999. Introduction. *Daedalus* 128(4), vii–x.

Konrad, M. 2005. *Nameless Relations: Anonymity, Melanesia and Reproductive Gift Exchange between British Ova Donors and Recipients*. Oxford: Berghahn Books.

Kopytoff, I. 1986. The Cultural Biography of Things: Commoditization as Process. In *The Social Life of Things: Commodities in Cultural Perspective*, ed. A. Appadurai. Cambridge: Cambridge University Press.

Laidlaw, J. 2002. For an Anthropology of Ethics and Freedom. *Journal of the Royal Anthropological Institute* 8(2), 311–32.

————. 2014. *The Subject of Virtue: An Anthropology of Ethics and Freedom.* Cambridge: Cambridge University Press.

Lambek, M. 2008. Value and Virtue. *Anthropological Theory* 8(2), 133–57.

————, ed. 2010. *Ordinary Ethics: Anthropology, Language, and Action.* New York: Fordham University Press.

Lamoreaux, J. 2013. Infertile Futures: Sperm and Science in a Chinese Environment. Unpublished PhD thesis, University of California, San Francisco and University of California, Berkeley.

Layne, L. L. 1996. "How's the Baby Doing?" Struggling with Narratives of Progress in a Neonatal Intensive Care Unit. *Medical Anthropology Quarterly* 10(4), 624–56.

Lee, E., J. Bristow, C. Faircloth, and J. Macvarish. 2014. *Parenting Culture Studies.* London: Palgrave Macmillan.

Little, J. 1997. Constructions of Rural Women's Voluntary Work. *Gender, Place & Culture* 4(2), 197–210.

Lutz, C. 1988. *Unnatural Emotions: Everyday Sentiments on a Micronesian Atoll and Their Challenge to Western Theory.* Chicago: University of Chicago Press.

Macdonald, S. 1997. *Reimagining Culture: Histories, Identities, and the Gaelic Renaissance.* Oxford: Berg.

Mackie, J. 2012. *Pearl Diving by Moonlight*, ed. K. Murray. Aberdeen: Malfranteaux Concepts.

Macnaghten, P., and J. Urry. 1998. *Contested Natures.* London: Sage.

Markens, S. 2007. *Surrogate Motherhood and the Politics of Reproduction.* Berkeley: University of California Press.

Martin, E. 2001. *The Woman in the Body: A Cultural Analysis of Reproduction.* Boston: Beacon Press.

Mattingly, C. 2014. *Moral Laboratories: Family Peril and the Struggle for a Good Life.* Berkeley: University of California Press.

Mauss, M. 2002. *The Gift.* Abingdon: Routledge.

Milton, K. ed. 1993. *Environmentalism: The View from Anthropology.* London: Routledge.

Minke Whale Escapes from Harbour. 2007. BBC News Online, 3 August. http://news.bbc.co.uk/1/hi/scotland/north_east/6927296.stm.

Mol, A., I. Moser, and J. Pols, eds. 2010. *Care in Practice: On Tinkering in Clinics, Homes and Farms.* Bielefeld: transcript.

Momus. 2009. *The Book of Scotlands.* Berlin: Sternberg Press.

Moore, K., K. Inez McGuire, R. Gordon, and T. J. Woodruff. 2011. Birth Control Hormones in Water: Separating Myth from Fact. *Contraception* 84:115–18.

Moray Firth Partnership. n.d. Moray Firth Special Area of Conservation. http://www.morayfirth-partnership.org/sac.html.

Morini, C. 2014. The Feminization of Labour in Cognitive Capitalism. *Feminist Review* 87:40–59.

Mulkay, M. 1997. *The Embryo Research Debate: Science and the Politics of Reproduction.* Cambridge: Cambridge University Press.

Nadel-Klein, J. 2003. *Fishing for Heritage: Modernity and Loss along the Scottish Coast.* New York: Berg.

Nalder, I. 2000. *Scotland's Golf in Days of Steam.* Dalkeith: Scottish Cultural Press.

National Institute of Environmental Health Sciences. 2010. *Endocrine Disruptors.* National Institutes of Health. https://www.niehs.nih.gov/health /materials/endocrine_disruptors_508.pdf.

National Records of Scotland. Scotland's Census—Area Profiles. http:// www.scotlandscensus.gov.uk/ods-web/area.html.

O'Riordan, T. 1981. *Environmentalism.* London: Pion.

Oakley, A. 1986. *From Here to Maternity: Becoming a Mother.* London: Penguin.

Pande, A. 2009. Not an "Angel," Not a "Whore": Surrogates as "Dirty" Workers in India. *Indian Journal of Gender Studies* 16(2), 141–73.

———. 2014. "At Least I Am Not Sleeping with Anyone": Resisting the Stigma of Commercial Surrogacy in India. *Feminist Studies* 36(2), 292–312.

Parry, J. 1986. The Gift, the Indian Gift and the "Indian Gift." *Man,* n.s., 21(3), 453–73.

Parry, J., and M. Bloch, eds. 1989. *Money and the Morality of Exchange.* Cambridge: Cambridge University Press.

Parsons, E.C.M. 2012. From Whaling to Whale Watching: A History of Cetaceans in Scotland. *The Glasgow Naturalist* 25(4). http://www.glasgownaturalhistory.org.uk/gn25_4/parsons.pdf.

Paxson, H. 2004. *Making Modern Mothers: Ethics and Family Planning in Urban Greece.* Berkeley: University of California Press.

———. 2013. *The Life of Cheese: Crafting Food and Value in America.* Berkeley: University of California Press.

Pedwell, C. 2014. *Affective Relations: The Transnational Politics of Empathy.* London: Palgrave Macmillan.

Petchesky, R. P. 1987. Fetal Images: The Power of Visual Culture in the Politics of Reproduction. *Feminist Studies* 13(2), 263–92.

Pfeffer, N. 1993. *The Stork and the Syringe: Political History of Reproductive Medicine.* New York: Wiley.

Pike, S. M. 2001. *Earthly Bodies, Magical Selves: Contemporary Pagans and the Search for Community.* Berkeley: University of California Press.

Power, N. 2009. *One Dimensional Woman.* Ropley: o Books.

Puig de la Bellacasa, M. 2010. Ethical Doings in Naturecultures. *Ethics, Place & Environment: A Journal of Philosophy & Geography* 13(2), 151–69.

———. 2012. "Nothing Comes without Its World": Thinking with Care. *Sociological Review* 60(2), 197–216.

Radkau, J. 2014. *The Age of Ecology.* Cambridge: Polity Press.

Ragoné, H. 1994. *Surrogate Motherhood: Conception in the Heart.* Boulder, CO: Westview Press.

Rapp, R. 1999. *Testing Women, Testing the Fetus: The Social Impact of Amniocentesis in America.* London: Routledge.

Rapport, N. 1993. *Diverse World Views in an English Village.* Edinburgh University Press.

———. 2010. The Ethics of Participant Observation. In *The Ethnographic Self as Resource: Writing Memory and Experience into Ethnography,* ed. P. Collins and A. Gallinat, 78–94. Oxford: Berghahn Books.

Rayment, Juliet. 2014. Emotional Labour: A Story of Midwifery Research. Paper given at "Researching Human Reproduction: Methodological and Ethical Aspects," De Montfort University, 5 December.

Robbins, J. 2012. On Becoming Ethical Subjects: Freedom, Constraint, and the Anthropology of Morality. *Anthropology of This Century.* http://aotcpress .com/articles/ethical-subjects-freedom-constraint-anthropology -morality/.

Roberts, C. 2007. *Messengers of Sex: Hormones, Biomedicine and Feminism.* Cambridge: Cambridge University Press.

Roberts, E.F.S. 1998. "Native" Narratives of Connectedness: Surrogate Motherhood and Technology. In *Cyborg Babies: From Techno-Sex to Techno-Tots,* ed. R. E. Davis-Floyd and J. Dumit. New York: Routledge.

Satz, D. 1992. Markets in Women's Reproductive Labor. *Philosophy and Public Affairs* 21(2), 107–31.

Schneider, D. 1968. *American Kinship: A Cultural Account.* Chicago: University of Chicago Press.

———. 1984. *A Critique of the Study of Kinship.* Ann Arbor: University of Michigan Press.

Scotch Whisky Association. 2011. Scotch Whisky Association. Briefing for the new Scottish Parliament. June.

Scott, D. N. 2009. "Gender-Benders": Sex and Law in the Constitution of Polluted Bodies. *Feminist Legal Studies* 17(3), 241–65.

Scott, N. J., and E.C.M. Parsons. 2005. A Survey of Public Opinion in Southwest Scotland on Cetacean Conservation Issues. *Aquatic Conservation* 15:299–312.

Scottish Government. 2007. *Report of the Review of Infertility Services in Scotland.* Edinburgh: Scottish Government. http://www.scotland.gov.uk /Publications/2007/03/28103201/1.

———. 2010. *Demographic Change in Scotland.* Edinburgh: Scottish Government. http://www.scotland.gov.uk/Publications/2010/11/24111237/6.

———. 2013. *NHS IVF Services to Be Fairer and Faster*. Edinburgh: Scottish Government.

Shelley, M. W. 2003. *Frankenstein, or, The Modern Prometheus*. London: Penguin.

Slaughter, S. R., R. Hearns-Stokes, T. van der Vlugt, and H. V. Joffe. 2014. FDA Approval of Doxylamine-Pyridoxine Therapy for Use in Pregnancy. *New England Journal of Medicine* 370(12), 1081–83.

Spallone, P., and D. L. Steinberg. 1987. *Made to Order: The Myth of Reproductive and Genetic Progress*. Oxford: Pergamon Press.

Stanworth, M. 1991. *Reproductive Technologies: Gender, Motherhood and Medicine*. New York: Wiley.

Stoett, P. J. 1997. *The International Politics of Whaling*. Vancouver: UBC Press.

Strathern, M. 1980. No Nature, No Culture: The Hagen Case. In *Nature, Culture and Gender*, ed. C. P. MacCormack and M. Strathern. Cambridge: Cambridge University Press.

———. 1981. *Kinship at the Core: An Anthropology of Elmdon, a Village in North-west Essex in the Nineteen-Sixties*. Cambridge: Cambridge University Press.

———. 1988. *The Gender of the Gift: Problems with Women and Problems with Society in Melanesia*. Berkeley: University of California Press.

———. 1992a. *After Nature: English Kinship in the Late Twentieth Century*. Cambridge: Cambridge University Press.

———. 1992b. *Reproducing the Future: Essays on Anthropology, Kinship and the New Reproductive Technologies*. Manchester: Manchester University Press.

———. 2003. Surrogacy: Still Giving Nature a Helping Hand? In *Surrogate Motherhood: International Perspectives*, ed. R. Cook, S. D. Sclater, and F. Kaganas, 281–96. Oxford: Hart Publishing.

Subtitle Decision "Puzzles" Scots. 2006. BBC News Online, 4 August. http://news.bbc.co.uk/1/hi/entertainment/5244738.stm.

Suizzo, A.-M. 2004. Mother-Child Relationships in France: Balancing Autonomy and Affiliation in Everyday Interactions. *Ethos* 32(3), 293–323.

Taylor, J. S. 1998. Image of Contradiction: Obstetrical Ultrasound in American Culture. In *Reproducing Reproduction: Kinship, Power, and Technological Innovation*, ed. S. Franklin and H. Ragoné. Philadelphia: University of Pennsylvania Press.

Taylor, M. 2008. *Living Working Countryside: The Taylor Review*. London: Department for Communities and Local Government.

Teman, E. 2010. *Birthing a Mother: The Surrogate Body and the Pregnant Self*. Berkeley: University of California Press.

Thompson, C. 2001. Strategic Naturalizing: Kinship in an Infertility Clinic. In *Relative Values: Reconfiguring Kinship Studies*. Durham, NC: Duke University Press.

———. 2002. When Elephants Stand for Competing Models of Nature. In *Complexities: Social Studies of Knowledge Practices*, ed. J. Law and A. Mol. Durham, NC: Duke University Press.

———. 2005. *Making Parents: The Ontological Choreography of Reproductive Technologies*. Cambridge, MA: MIT Press.

———. 2013. *Good Science: The Ethical Choreography of Stem Cell Research*. Cambridge, MA: MIT Press.

Titmuss, R. M. 1997. *The Gift Relationship: From Human Blood to Social Policy*. London: LSE Books.

Trubek, A. B. 2008. *The Taste of Place: A Cultural Journey into Terroir*. Berkeley: University of California Press.

Trump to Build New Clubhouse Despite Wind Farm Row. 2014. *The Scotsman*, 7 August. http://www.scotsman.com/news/scotland/top-stories/trump-to-build-new-clubhouse-despite-wind-farm-row-1-3501709.

Tutton, R. 2002. Gift Relationships in Genetics Research. *Science as Culture* 11(4), 523–42.

Van Dooren, T. 2014. Care. *Environmental Humanities* 5(2), 291–94.

Wall, G. 2001. Moral Constructions of Motherhood in Breastfeeding Discourse. *Gender and Society* 15(4), 592–610.

Warnock, M. 1985a. *A Question of Life: The Warnock Report on Human Fertilisation and Embryology*. Oxford: Blackwell.

———. 1985b. Moral Thinking and Government Policy : The Warnock Committee on Human Embryology. *The Millbank Memorial Fund Quarterly: Health and Society* 63(3), 504–22.

Watson, M. 2003. *Being English in Scotland: Population, Space and Place*. Edinburgh: Edinburgh University Press.

Weston, K. 1998. Forever Is a Long Time: Romancing the Real in Gay Kinship Ideologies. In *Long Slow Burn: Sexuality and Social Science*. London: Routledge.

———. 2001. Kinship, Controversy, and the Sharing of Substance: The Race/Class Politics of Blood Transfusion. In *Relative Values: Reconfiguring Kinship Studies*, ed. S. Franklin and S. McKinnon. Durham, NC: Duke University Press.

Whitfield, N. 2013. Who Is My Stranger? Origins of the Gift in Wartime London, 1939–45. *Journal of the Royal Anthropological Institute* 19:S95–S117.

Wilkinson, S. 2003. *Bodies for Sale: Ethics and Exploitation in the Human Body Trade*. London: Routledge.

William Grant & Sons Breaks £1bn Turnover Barrier Again. 2013. *The Herald*, 30 September. http://www.heraldscotland.com/business/company-news/william-grant-sons-breaks-1bn-turnover-barrier-again.22300962.

Williams, R. 1975. *The Country and the City*. Oxford: Oxford University Press.

———. 1977. *Marxism and Literature*. Oxford: Oxford University Press.

————. 2004 [1974]. *Television: Technology and Cultural Form*. London: Routledge.

Wilson, D. 2011a. Creating the "Ethics Industry": Mary Warnock, in Vitro Fertilization and the History of Bioethics in Britain. *BioSocieties* 6(2), 121–41.

————. 2011b. Who Guards the Guardians? Ian Kennedy, Bioethics and the "Ideology of Accountability" in British Medicine. *Social History of Medicine* 25(1), 193–211.

————. 2013. What Can History Do for Bioethics? *Bioethics* 27(4), 215–23.

————. 2014. *The Making of British Bioethics*. Manchester: Manchester University Press.

Wolfram, S. 1989. Surrogacy in the United Kingdom. In *New Approaches to Human Reproduction: Social and Ethical Dimensions*, ed. L. M. Whiteford and M. L. Poland. Boulder, CO: Westview Press.

Yanagisako, S., and C. Delaney, eds. 2013. *Naturalizing Power: Essays in Feminist Cultural Analysis*. New York: Routledge.

Zelizer, V.A.R. 1997. *The Social Meaning of Money*. Princeton: Princeton University Press.

Zipper, J., and S. Sevenhuijsen. 1987. Surrogacy: Feminist Notions of Motherhood Reconsidered. In *Reproductive Technologies: Gender, Motherhood and Medicine*, ed. M. Stanworth. Cambridge: Polity Press.

INDEX

Aberdeen, 185

Aberdeenshire, 37, 64

abortion, ethics of, 12

Adopt a Dolphin, 75, 178–79; and the anthropomorphism of dolphins, 178–79; parents as adopters, 179; and the term "adoption," 179

adoption, 93

Ahmed, Sara, on emotions, 191

Almeling, Rene, 211n24

altruism, 150; and blood donation, 175–76; and parenting, 69; and surrogacy, 48, 147, 150, 152–56; and women, 148

assisted reproductive technologies (ART), 7, 11–12, 150–51, 194, 197; and ambivalence, 94–95, 158, 192; and concerns about kinship, 94–95; and context, 156–58; and the decision not to have children, 9–10; and "designer babies," 95, 188, 207n20; feminist criticism of, 10; and human endangerment, 170; inequalities in access to in the UK, 8–9; and the medicalisation of reproduction and infertility, 9; and parenthood as chosen and planned, 66; and people's creation of children "of their own," 160; and the "plight of the infertile couple" trope, 149; and pressure on infertile people, 9; promissory value of, 98; public and media debate about, 8, 18, 152; and the

selection of traits, 212n9; the transnational ART industry, 212n9

attachment theory, 120

Basu, Paul: on roots tourists to Scotland, 36; on the "Scottish diaspora," 211n36

Baxter, Anthony, 214n3

Becker, Gay, on infertile American couples, 67

Bell, Ann V., on inequalities in access to ART, 8

Bendectin, 113, 115, 209n6; brand names of (Debendox and Diclegis), 209n6

bioethics, 13; "empirical turn" of, 16; inherent individualism in, 15; and the issue of payment or compensation for bodily "products" and "services," 13; and the prioritisation of principles over practices, 15; and questions of universalism versus particularism, 14–15; shaping of by context, 16–17

biotechnology industry, 9

Blair, Tony, 37

blood donation, 174–78; and altruism, 175–76; and the anonymous recipient, 213n23; blood as the carrier of kinship, 176; blood as partible from its original body, 176; ethics of, 178; in the UK, 213n23

Bonaccorso, Monica, 211n41

Bowlby, John, 120